Your Ultimate Pilates Body® Challenge

Your Ultimate

Pilates Body® Challenge

at the gym, on the mat, and on the move

Brooke Siler

Broadway Books

New York

BROADWAY

Broadway Books titles may be purchased for business or promotional use or for special sales. For information, please write to: Special Markets Department, Random House, Inc., 1745 Broadway, New York, NY 10019.

DISCLAIMER: The instructions and advice in this book are in no way intended as a substitute for medical counseling. We advise the reader to consult with his/her doctor before beginning this or any other exercise regimen. The author and the publisher disclaim any liability or loss, personal or otherwise, resulting from the exercises in this book.

PRINTED IN THE UNITED STATES OF AMERICA

BROADWAY BOOKS and its logo, a letter B bisected on the diagonal, are trademarks of Random House, Inc.

Visit our Web site at www.broadwaybooks.com

First edition published 2006

Book design by Ruth Lee-Mui
Illustrated by Meredith Hamilton
Illustrations on page 18 by Jackie Aher
Photographs by Marc Royce
Photo on page 7 appears courtesy of Sean Gallagher and The New York Pilates Studio®. For more information go to www.pilates-studio.com

Library of Congress Cataloging-in-Publication Data

Siler, Brooke, 1968–
Your ultimate Pilates body : at the gym, on the mat, and on the move / Brooke Siler.
p. cm.
1. Pilates method. 2. Swiss exercise balls. I. Title.

RA781.4.S55 2006
613.7'1—dc22
2005047135

ISBN 0-7679-1982-3

1 3 5 7 9 10 8 6 4 2

Pilates Body® and Brooke Siler's Pilates studio in New York, re:AB®, are registered trademarks. Invisible Workout™ is trademarked.

I would like to dedicate this book to my magical February 24th boys,

MEVIN AND **SEBASTIAN**.

What a difference a day makes.

contents

Your Ultimate Pilates Body® Challenge

Welcome to Your
Ultimate Pilates Body® Challenge!

As many of you know, Pilates is one of those wonderful phenomena that has broken through the surface of the collective consciousness in the last few years to emerge as a "hot new trend." Fewer people realize that Pilates brings almost one hundred years of history with it.

Created by Joseph H. Pilates to strengthen his frail and sickly body, Pilates was then translated to specific apparatus to help those unable to support their own body weight. It debuted in 1920s New York City as the lengthening, strengthening, and rehabilitation secret of stars, starlets, dancers, and acrobats and then all but disappeared for the next few decades, remaining known only to the small population interested in physical fitness. Today that demographic extends to include most everyone looking for strong, long, lean muscles, inspired either by the media culture or touched by an injury.

Dressed up or dressed down, at the core of the Pilates movement today still beats the heart of the Pilates of yesteryear. Designed to use the art and science of muscle control—what Joseph Pilates termed *Contrology*—to help you achieve the body that looks good, feels good, and sustains you for a lifetime, Pilates is ageless, colorless, and genderless; and once incorporated into your subconscious, it marries the joy of movement with the efficiency of your most challenging workout.

> Correctly executed and mastered to the point of subconscious reaction, these exercises will reflect grace and balance in your routine activities. Contrology exercises build a sturdy body and sound mind capable of performing everyday tasks with ease and perfection. They

also provide tremendous reserve energy for sports, recreation and emergencies.

(Return to Life through Contrology, Joseph H. Pilates)

Many of you are old friends, readers I know from *The Pilates Body*. I hope, too, many of you are new friends, readers who have picked up *Your Ultimate Pilates Body Challenge* because you are intrigued by expanding your awareness and your body's potential. And, finally, welcome to the reader who is not yet in shape—or who was in shape and is somehow, now, mysteriously, feeling as if he or she were living in someone else's body, because I can relate! Halfway through the writing of this book, I had a baby—and suddenly became my own audience. So, as I wrote and rewrote, read and reread this book's philosophy I also relived the work from the ground up.

I began writing *Your Ultimate Pilates Body Challenge* before I was pregnant. Why? Because I was seeing what I felt was an alarming trend. Every day I had clients coming in and doing amazing work, then abandoning basic posture and alignment before they got to the sidewalk. I began to do some research. What I discovered was a twofold problem: Clients were stagnating within their solo workout sessions, and they weren't applying what they had learned in the studio when they were off the mat. Off the mat? Yes. Because Pilates is more than the exercises performed in a studio. It's about personal responsibility, active self-care, and feeling good as you move through your day and your life. More than a series of movements, it's a philosophy and a mindset. Because, if your brain is not active and engaged and working, it won't matter how good you look; you won't feel your best. Without your conscious brain, your body is like any piece of equipment without an owner's manual. Usable, but too often a mystery.

And, as I said, I understand that feeling of mystery! After having my beautiful baby, I discovered that even though I had been physically fit, and educated, my body had become a mystery. Although I knew intellectually where I should be lifting from and which muscles I should be engaging, the communication lines between my brain and my body appeared to have been disconnected. I needed to reread the owner's manual. So, *Your Ultimate Pilates Body Challenge* became that manual. *Your Ultimate Pilates Body Challenge* asks you to take a real look at your body—beyond the number that appears on the scale. Can you discover why you've hit a plateau within your workout? Why you always end up with knee pain? Why your neck feels strained at the end of the day?

I want you to get moving—and have fun and *be efficient* while doing what you do. One thing I've learned as a new mom is that time is of the essence; I needed to get more out of less time. *Your Ultimate Pilates Body Challenge* is full of both new mat routines and ways to take what you've learned in the studio off the mat and into the world with the Pilates-Conscious Cardio Circuit at the Gym, the Invisible Workout™, and Pilates for the Sports-Minded.

People need three things out of their fitness programs:

- Strength
- Flexibility
- Cardiovascular conditioning

Pilates has all three! Too often, however, it is thought of as a system that is specific to dancers, rehabilitation, or meditation.

I wrote *Your Ultimate Pilates Body Challenge* to help Pilates beat this rap, to change the perception that Pilates is limited to an arena outside your daily scope of living or working out. Like many of you, I am busy multitasking the many matters that make up my day-to-day life; and when I am ready, willing, and able to work out, it can't be so complicated as to put me off, so boring as to not challenge me, or so ineffectual as to waste my precious time. With those principles in mind, I put together the building blocks of *Your Ultimate Pilates Body Challenge* so that they can be stacked and moved around as best suit your needs.

With the principles you'll find in *Your Ultimate Pilates Body Challenge,* those of you just beginning can create a safe, challenging, and efficient workout, and those of you who have become bored with your routine can infuse an old workout with renewed energy and purpose. Interval challenges are included to enhance your cardiovascular output and help burn more calories and dissolve fat.

When you're in the gym, I'll teach you to use your Pilates principles to turn a stale workout routine into a fat-burning, muscle-producing, *efficient* use of your time. No more plugging away for hours on the same old course, stomping up the same hills, or hanging over the same handlebars.

As a self-confessed gym junkie, I was compelled to create the Pilates-Conscious Cardio Circuit. Armed with the information in *Your Ultimate Pilates Body Challenge,* you will be able to complete a Pilates-aware circuit at the gym on a variety of machines that will burn more calories in less time. Once you have completed the circuit, you can hit your mat for a 10- to 20-minute Pilates mat routine while your heart is still pumping in the target zone. Fast, fun, and extremely challenging, the Pilates-Conscious Cardio Circuit is a high-powered, superconscious workout that engages you both mentally and physically.

For my fellow die-hard Pilates Matwork fans *Your Ultimate Pilates Body Challenge* is chock full of new movements, engaging visual and verbal metaphors, tips to progress or modify your matwork, and four fantastic body-specific programs. Adding Abs, Lean Lower Body, Perfecting Posture, and Finding Flexibility contain both the fun and the challenges you need to target your main areas of concern while still giving yourself a total-body workout.

Athletes and sports fans alike will gain insight into their game from the information in the sports section. Here, I took the principles of Pilates and applied them to four of the sports so many of us know and love: tennis, golf, skiing, and snowboarding. As you begin to incorporate this information, you'll add depth and proficiency to your game. Every great athlete must combine artistry with technique, form with function. Pilates is steeped in the art and science of body movement/physiology and a few great visual cues or Pilates form tips can be the difference between good and great when it counts. Whatever your sport of choice is, the guidelines of this section apply.

But what about the days when you can't get to the gym or hit the courts, the course, or the slopes? Unique to *Your Ultimate Pilates Body Challenge* is my Invisible Workout, which will serve to keep you tuned in and toned up throughout the day by using simple Pilates-conscious moves that you can execute anywhere and everywhere. Whether a handbag or a hand weight, a child or a chest press—the Invisible Workout will teach you to use the world around you as a tool for improving your fitness and physique.

The Invisible Workout helps you incorporate basic Pilates principles into your daily activities, making the world your gym as well as your oyster. Before my son was born, I had the misguided assumption that I would snap back into shape with little to no effort at all. My Pilates practice served me incredibly well throughout the entire pregnancy, and there was no reason to believe anything but a miraculous recovery was in store. What a rude awakening to discover that my body had a different game plan. I am thankful I had *Your Ultimate Pilates*

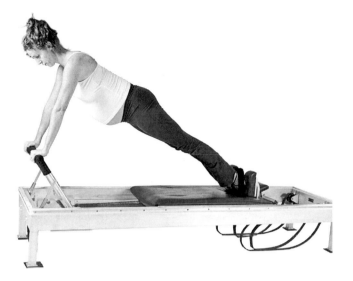

Body Challenge to work on. Every activity and movement in my daily life became another chance to regain my strength and control over my body. Although they seemed like baby steps at times, they added up to more.

The Invisible Workout asks if you can learn to apply the fundamentals of Pilates to real-life situations. For everything from taking out the garbage to sinking a hole-in-one. What will it mean when you can? It will mean you will be working your body naturally throughout the entire day, instead of working your body inefficiently for 1 or 2 hours every other day at the gym. Becoming observant, training the body from the inside out, beginning to rely on its deepest muscles to sit and stand and walk properly, means not only carrying and lifting but running, skating, swimming . . . all your favorite activities begin to flow with

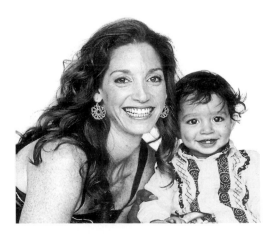

ease and efficiency. One of the ways I know my work with clients is starting to pay off is they come in with observations about how they have begun to sit or stand or jog differently, with awareness, and how much better this has made them feel throughout the day. This tells me that they have begun to realize that fitness is not something to put on with their sweat socks—fitness has become second nature, a way of being as they move through the world. What will that translate into? Pounds melting away. Why? Because incorporating these principles into everyday activities means constantly working the body intelligently. And a constant workout needs more muscle. And muscle burns more calories than fat. All of which raises your metabolism, and voilà! a supremely toned and shapelier you.

One of the things I've discovered is helpful in this process is to use what I call *Metaforms:* visual images, or metaphors, that will remind you of your best body form. That's why I've provided visuals throughout the book that will make your brain your best coach. Think of your brain as a muscle—the strongest you've got.

I've also included challenges in each section to help keep brain and body engaged as you move forward. Some of you will take to these immediately, some of you will get there soon—we all define challenge differently.

Your Ultimate Pilates Body Challenge removes the need for excuses as to why you're not where you want to be physically. It jump starts the beginner and challenges the experienced. It removes the element of boredom because of its multifaceted design intended to mix and match exercises for any situation. This book works as hard as you do (or will) to make sure that your workout time is efficient, exciting, innovative, and ultimately produces the effects you desire.

Are you ready?

The Man,
the Method,
the Movement

the man

Before we begin, a word about the man himself, Joseph Pilates, who has done so much to influence so many people's lives.

Joseph H. Pilates was born in Germany in 1880. A sickly child, he suffered from asthma, rheumatic fever, and rickets. Having a father who was a gymnast, and a mother who was a naturopath, ill-health wasn't his destiny, however. He began studying anatomy in textbooks and in life—hiding in the woods for hours to watch the movements of the animals. He also studied yoga and Zen meditation. By the age of fourteen, he had developed his physique to the point that he was modeling for anatomy charts. He went on to become an accomplished gymnast and boxer.

During World War I, he was interned in England. While working in a hospital as an orderly, he noticed that many patients recovered more quickly if they were given exercises to do. Because many of them were incredibly weak, he devised a number of exercises that made use of the bedsprings for resistance. This is the foundation of one of his more famous pieces of equipment, the Cadillac. Ultimately, his series of exercises numbered approximately five hundred. He named it "Contrology," and defined it as "complete coordination of body, mind and spirit." The exercises focused on developing the core stabilizing muscles of the abdomen, or powerhouse, which frees the rest of the body for greater mobility and flexibility—ensuring everything is working at its best.

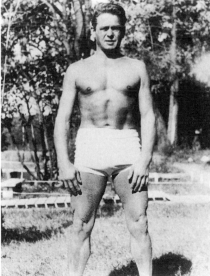

the method

The last few years of fitness fads have left us craving something with staying power. While other fitness trends may lack longevity, Pilates has been practiced for almost a century. Joseph Pilates developed his method in the early 1900s, and today it's going stronger than ever. Why? Because it's based on solid physiological methodology, not gimmicks. This section looks at a couple of Pilates's principles that support the ongoing Pilates challenge:

Taking responsibility: Pilates believed that you have a personal responsibility for your health that extends beyond an hour's workout. Incorporating Pilates's principles into every area of your life brings your fitness awareness to another level and subsequently allows everything you do to contribute to your well-being and, consequently, your self-esteem. When you're off the mat, or out of Invisible Workout mode, you can still do more: Is there some health research you've been meaning to do? Eating habits that you've been wanting to incorporate? A fitness class you've been meaning to try? The responsibility for your health begins with you.

Your mind is a muscle! The concept behind the challenges and Metaforming: Pilates believed that it is as important for your mind to be engaged as it is for your powerhouse to be engaged. In other words, mind *and* body, not mind *or* body. Pilates learned from everyone and everything around him. For example, one of Pilates's mandates was to watch how animals move: their economy of motion, their seeming effortlessness, their total-body control, their ability to stay injury free. I challenge you to do the same: What can we take away from their innate intelligence? Similar challenges appear in special "Challenge" sections throughout the book, which are designed to take your mental and physical workout to the next level. I have also employed a fail-safe way to add enjoyment while boosting the efficiency of your workouts through my system of creative visualization: Metaforming.

my method: metaforming

Using our minds creatively is a power we all possess, yet exercise infrequently. I have found that when I use creative visual metaphors to highlight the essence of the exercises, clients' bodies conform faster to proper physiological form. Hence the concept of Metaforming.

As the child of incredibly intuitive parents, and a father who taught me to "think warm" on the coldest of days, I was destined to use creativity in my Pilates practice. In fact, my older brother, Todd Siler, took creative thinking to its ultimate degree by developing an entire educational system with the metaphor as its central theme (www.thinklikeagenius.com). Whereas Todd has employed the meta*phor* I now wish to formally introduce the meta*form:* the mental use of visual and verbal metaphor to spur the body to achieve proper form.

By using the visual metaphors your body will respond faster to the task at hand. If I tell you to "use the contraction of your abdominal muscles to stabilize the muscles of your spine" as you perform an exercise, you may very well be able to do that. However, if I tell you to "imagine you have a corset cinched around your waist securing your center," chances are that you will not only employ more muscles to create the feeling of what you imagine but will also use the muscles with proper form. This inevitably creates a more efficient, effective use of your workout time.

Now I know some of you may be asking, "What if I'm not a creative or imaginative person?" You soon will be. I have provided hundreds of visual and verbal references to get you started. Remember, the more you exercise your mind to think creatively the better at it you will become.

More isn't better, better is better: Pilates believed in working smarter, not longer. As he said, "Never do 10 pounds of effort for a 5-pound movement." This is the same principle behind the Pilates-Conscious Cardio Circuit and Pilates Matwork routines.

We've all heard people boasting about how much time they've spent on the treadmill, or climbing endless stairs to nowhere. With the Pilates-Conscious Cardio Circuit—because you are moving with awareness from the get-go—you don't have to keep on and on. You burn more calories in a shorter amount of time, which means you can be leaving the gym for a guilt-free dinner and a movie, while others are still spinning their wheels.

Engaging your powerhouse to lengthen, strengthen, and disengage from your pain: Pilates believed in training the body to move with grace and efficiency all the time. To that end, the Pilates secret is, and always has been, the powerhouse—which in today's vernacular has become known as your "core." In days of yore, when the Charles Atlases of the world were advocating strengthening your core through thickening or compressing your center to secure your low back, Joseph Pilates recognized that the internal organs housed within that area were being compromised.

> [Slouching] upsets the equilibrium of the body resulting in disarrangement of various organs, including the bones and muscles as well as the nerves, blood vessels and glands. . . . [P]roper carriage of the spine is the only natural way to prevent against abdominal obesity, shortness of breath, asthma, high and low blood pressure and various forms of heart disease.
>
> (*Your Health,* Joseph H. Pilates)

By strengthening these core/powerhouse muscles and using that strength to help lengthen the surrounding muscles, many things are achieved: Posture is improved by strengthening the stabilizing muscles of the spine; digestion and *circulation* are improved through the newfound length and space around the internal organs; the waistline is slimmed; and, whether or not weight loss is your goal, your clothes will begin to feel loose around your middle. In essence, contracting your abdominal muscles, lifting them in and up your spine, will serve to become the new state of awareness within your body and anything less will feel uncomfortable, tired, or sloppy. You will learn to use your lungs to breathe laterally in such as way so as not to disturb the secure foundation of your engaged powerhouse. While this may seem hopeful at best to you now, it will soon be as natural as taking the breath itself. By simultaneously contracting our abdominal muscles as we lengthen our spines, we create a strong foundation—built to withstand the weight of our body throughout the tasks of our day. By using our power centers, we eliminate wasted energy, inefficient and potentially dangerous movements, and a flabby tummy all at once.

the movement

Pilates referred to his method as the Art of Contrology: the study and science of controlled, considered movement. Regardless of the activity, some similar elements always remain in play—stability/mobility, resistance/opposition, leverage, articulation, balance. Familiarizing yourself with these, along with the eight guiding principles of *Your Ultimate Pilates Body Challenge,* will ensure that no matter what you are doing you are applying Pilates's workout-enhancing principles: They are the foundation on which all the method is laid.

THE EIGHT GUIDING PRINCIPLES OF *YOUR ULTIMATE PILATES BODY CHALLENGE*

Concentration: It is your mind that wills your body to work; therefore, pay attention to the movements you perform and how your muscles respond to the attention.

Control: True muscle control means no sloppy or haphazard movements.

Center: There is a large group of muscles making up our centers—our abdominals, low back, hips, and buttocks—that are termed the powerhouse in Pilates. All energy for the movements of Pilates initiates from the powerhouse and radiates to the extremities.

Precision: To leave out any detail of a specific movement is to lose the intrinsic value of the exercise. Therefore, choose to focus on doing a single precise and perfect movement over many half-hearted ones.

Breath: By employing full inhalations and full exhalations, you are expelling stale air and noxious gases from the depths of your lungs and replenishing your body with fresh air to energize and revitalize your system.

Fluidity: Dynamic, energetic movements replace the isolated and static or quick and jerky movements of other techniques. A focus on grace and economy of motion is emphasized over speed, and ultimately the movements should feel as fluid as a long stride or a waltz.

Imagination: It is the body that follows the will of the mind; therefore, using verbal and visual metaphors to create perceived resistance will increase efficiency and results.

Intuition: Listen to your body! It *does* know best.

stability/mobility

In essence, something moves while something else stays in place. Imagine a spring-loaded door (as on your refrigerator or oven). When you open that door the refrigerator itself stays still; it is stabilized by its weight. This stabilization allows for the mobility of the door. If the whole fridge moved as you tried to open the door, you wouldn't ever get to those leftovers! Well the body works in a similar fashion—that is, the more effectively you can stabilize one part of your body, the more efficiently the moving part will work to achieve the goal.

The Double Straight Leg Stretch is a great example of this concept in action. The goal of this stretch is to sufficiently stabilize the torso, through the powerhouse, to allow the legs to move freely in the hip joints. It is in fact the act of stabilizing the torso that triggers the correct powerhouse muscles to work and diminishes the need to grip through the leg muscles. Most people looking at this exercise might think that it was meant to work only your legs, as it's the

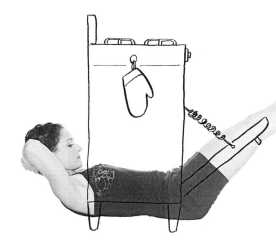

leg muscles that are engaged and moving. But what makes Pilates so efficient is what you don't see working; the upper, middle, and lower back; the abdominals; the buttocks; and even a good bit of neck and arm strength to help counterbalance the weight of the legs as they are lowered. This is why, performed correctly, the exercises of Pilates work every muscle in the body from the tips of your fingers to the tips of your toes.

resistance/opposition

Resistance and opposition are quite possibly the most important elements of all for achieving the potential length, strength, and stretch of the Pilates body. It is the power of a body as it acts in opposition to the pressure of another force.

Picture stretching a rubber band as if you were about to shoot it across the room. The stretching action works only if the two "ends" of it are being pulled away from each other. In other words, if you try to pull a rubber band with one finger and do not attach the other end to something stable, it won't stretch, you'll just be moving the rubber band through space. The body works in a similar fashion—that is, if you pull two of its parts away from each other you'll feel the stretch. To add to this equation, the more resistance you create with your muscles pulling in two different directions, the more stretch you'll achieve and the harder the muscles work.

Take the Roll Up as an example of creating resistance and opposition. We know that when reaching forward for your toes, an automatic stretch is created. What you may not know, however, is that the resistance you can create from your powerhouse will enhance that stretch and strengthen your muscles si-

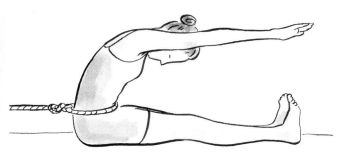

multaneously. For example, if you imagine being pulled back in your center as you try to stretch forward, instead of merely hanging over your thighs, you can create a greater stretch with more muscles engaged.

The Biceps Curls with the band on p. 67 is a great example of creating resistance with a rubber band. We know that by standing on one end of the band while pulling up on the other there is an automatic resistance that is created. What you may not know, however, is that if you imagine resistance as the band is lowered, the muscle elongates as it works. Of course, simply releasing the upward force on the band will return it to its starting position, but that doesn't require any work on your part—and that's just not Pilates.

Taking it a step further, learn to create resistance where there is none. That is, remove the band entirely but create the same force of resistance as if it were still there. I often tell clients that their muscles don't know the difference between a 10-pound dumbbell and 10 pounds of imagined resistance. The muscles will react to whatever your mind tells them is there. Using this creative tool throughout your workout is what creates the length and stretch of an active muscle, and it requires the will of your mind over your body.

leverage

Two forces that act in parallel and opposite directions create leverage. Imagine slowly pulling on the ends of a wishbone. The tension that is created from that pull is manifested in the center of the wishbone. Now apply that to your body as it is "pulled" in parallel and opposite directions, as in the exercise called Teaser III, when you are returning your body to the mat from the V position while simultaneously stretching out to full length.

If you simply lie back down, you will still have worked your stomach muscles a bit, but if you create leverage by reaching your arms and legs to opposite sides of the room and imagine you are being pulled, you will engage all the surrounding muscles as well as create length in your waist. As it's unlikely you'll ever have two actual forces pulling you in opposite directions, you will need to create this sensation by using the force of your imagination.

The Breathing exercise (p. 146) is also a great example of leverage: The resistance you need to create with your arms lowering is directly proportional to the force with which you raise your hips. If your arms come racing down without working as a lever to the lifting of the hips, you miss out on the ancillary benefit of toning your arms and also lose the control so integral to proper Pilates form.

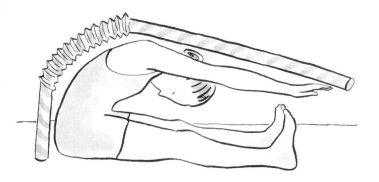

articulation

Articulation is the jointed connection of parts so that motion is possible.

A great example of this, and one I love to use, is the Spine Stretch Forward. Imagining your spine as a bendy straw is a near-perfect depiction of the ways in which you can visualize articulation so that you create a more effective exercise.

In the Spine Stretch Forward, while it is possible to effectively articulate your spine by simply bending forward, what we're looking for is the greatest amount of space you can put between each vertebra—each joint of the bendy straw, as it were—to lengthen the muscles of the spine and create breathing room for your organs. To achieve this, you must really use your powerhouse muscles and imagine yourself lifting up and over a large ball, or anything else that helps you feel the lengthening of your spine. From this position, try to roll your head down to the mat without losing any of the length or space between the vertebrae.

Not only is this more challenging but you'll find that proper articulation goes hand in hand with resistance and opposition in creating a longer, leaner more flexible you.

balance

Balance is the state of equilibrium between equal opposing forces. Let's call on the word *opposition* again and see how it figures into exercises requiring balance. Even though balance is required for what we consider to be the simple acts of walking and sitting, after toddlerhood most of us take it for granted because so few of our daily activities really challenge our balance. In Pilates, the exercises ask you to challenge the notion of balance being easy. In classic mat exercises, such as Rolling Like a Ball, Open Leg Rocker, and the Seal, you are asked to question and control the mus-

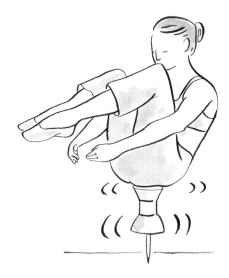

cles necessary for balance. Let's take the new challenge of the Stomach Massage I (p. 114) to dig a little deeper. While sitting on your tailbone, imagine shrinking the floor down to the size of a thumbtack and feel how much control your powerhouse needs to exert to ensure that the weight from another part of your body doesn't pull you off your seat. You will find that you are pulling your powerhouse in opposition to many muscles at once to achieve that state of balance. After a few more concentrated repetitions, you may have a whole new appreciation for standing upright!

a whole new you

Putting all of these elements together can lead to a phenomenal change in your body—and not just one that you feel, one that shows! Joseph Pilates was one of the first people to use "outcome studies." He'd take pictures of his clients when they began and then photograph them a few weeks later to show results. Today, before and after photos are a hallmark of every beauty magazine, but in Pilates's time, it was a revolutionary notion.

At re:AB® Pilates, my studio in New York City, we promise clients a new body in thirty sessions. Is this possible? Yes. And the same is true for you. If you commit to an exercise routine that engages your body, mind, and spirit for thirty sessions, I guarantee you will have an after photo that will make you proud.

Your
Amazing Body:
The Owner's Manual

As most of us who've taken the time to figure out our DVD players or program our cell phones know, sometimes it helps to have an idea of how a machine functions so that we can be aware of all the options at our command. Yet, when it comes to our body—the most high-tech piece of equipment we own—we rarely give the way it works a second thought. For many of us, this has led to the resigned conclusion that it isn't possible to change a body image that displeases us or to fix the chronic aches and pains that ail us. Not so! I believe the main reason for this apathy is that too often we are simply asked to be sheep, to accept wisdom and formulas handed down from so-called experts, rather than being encouraged to become our own expert. This chapter challenges you to start thinking about how to work from the inside out—to become the expert on your own body.

Looking at the anatomy drawings on pages 18 and 21 serves an important function. The University of Chicago did a study a few years ago on the power of visualization. A master group was divided into three sections. One section was taken to a basketball court and made to shoot free throws every day for 1 hour for one month. One section was asked to visualize shooting free throws for 1 hour a day for a month. The third section—the control group—did nothing. At the end of the month, the control group's average of baskets made had not changed; the group that had been physically shooting baskets had improved by 14 percent, and the group that had been visualizing shooting baskets had improved by 13 percent. In other words, being able to visualize where things are and how they work can go a long way toward helping you master the internal core muscles so integral to an understanding of the Pilates powerhouse.

By asking questions like, Why do I always end up with low back pain?

How can I work on improving my posture? How can I get more energy for my day?, you will begin to discover the minute movements that will cause a change in your physique.

mirror, mirror

In this section we'll look at your current state of health and postural habits. I've noticed that many clients have trouble doing an objective assessment of their bodies in the mirror, but this is the very best way to start your fitness program. With that information in hand, you can then target those areas you'd like to concentrate on going forward.

look through my eyes

When a client comes to see me they unknowingly begin their work as they walk in the door. My first inspiration comes from reading his or her body posture in its "natural" state and looking for anything that may stand out as imbalanced. These imbalances can contribute to almost all chronic ailments, including the purely aesthetic idea that "some articles may have shifted during flight."

I ask clients several questions to gain a better understanding of their bodies. Asking yourself these questions—and checking in your mirror to see if your answers are correct—can begin to shed light on where your alignment might be off.

After getting an idea of what you'll be working with on your own body, you'll be better adept at seeing the differences that clean lines and perfect posture make. From here you'll be prepared to tailor the work of each Challenge to your individual body's requirements.

Check all that apply to what you see in the mirror or know to be true about your body during a typical day:

❑ Do you habitually stand with your weight on one leg? Right or left?
❑ Do you habitually stand with your weight shifted into one hip? Right or left?
❑ Are you knocked-kneed? Bowlegged?
❑ Do you lock or even "hyperextend" your knees when you stand?
❑ Do you roll in or out on your feet? (You can check the heels of your shoes to see if they tend to wear out on one side or the other for the answer to this question.)

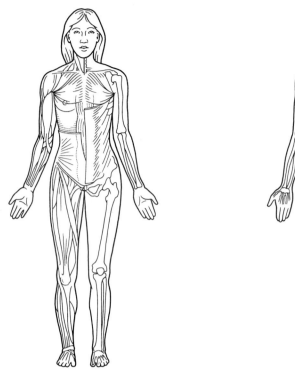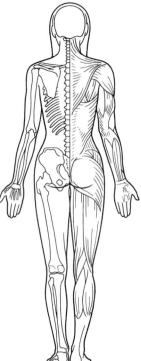

❑ Are your shoulders rounded forward?
❑ Is your chest lifted or concave?
❑ Does one shoulder appear higher than the other?
❑ Is your head habitually tilted in one way? Right or left? Forward or back?
❑ Is your back rounded? Upper, middle, or lower?
❑ Do you have a hollow/arched back when you stand? Upper or lower?
❑ Does your tummy protrude?

Did you stand taller or correct yourself as you made these assessments? If so, you are a step ahead in your journey to becoming your own best teacher.

If you've had trouble knowing what is correct or incorrect alignment or what constitutes healthy postural and breathing habits, the drawings above and the breathing and powerhouse exercises that follow will provide more informed answers.

the architecture of your body

We arrive in the world with all we need for a smoothly running machine. As we grow older, however, different physical habits cause some muscles to tighten and others to become weak, pulling our bones out of their natural alignment. This can result in everything from tennis elbow to lower back pain, to arthritis, which can occur when the body is out of structural balance, causing one joint to wear out before another. These drawings are simply to provide a quick visual reminder or reference point of the inherent elegance and efficiency of our structural foundation.

the many pluses of perfect posture

In addition to making you look taller and thinner and your clothes fit better, posture is the key to muscle and joint alignment and, in turn, to a healthy body. When we slouch, in addition to throwing off our natural balance, we crowd our internal organs—resulting in sluggish digestion, which can lead to problems from dull skin to a protruding "pooch" of a stomach and/or to overall weight gain. How can we begin to see where we are cheating? Is your body compensating? Torquing? Pinched? Twisted? Check these drawings, look in your mirror, ask a friend, compare and contrast.

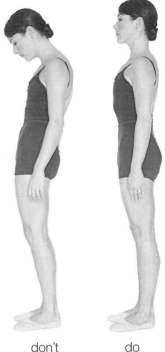

don't   do

the many bonuses of better breathing

Hearing that you need to learn to breathe correctly can be a bit like hearing that you need to learn to walk correctly . . . mysterious, if not irritating. The fact remains, however, that many of us do not maximize the potential created by better breathing—it truly can improve your exercise stamina and flush astonishing amounts of toxins from your system.

What you will notice as you begin breathing correctly is that in addition to being able to exercise longer and

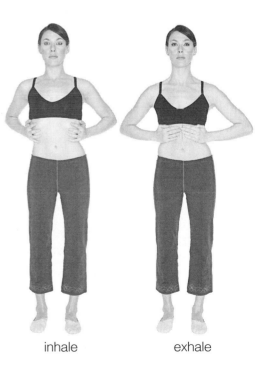

inhale   exhale

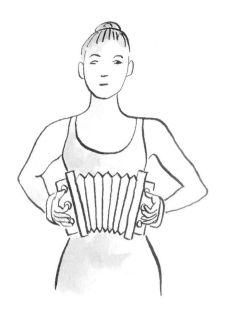

harder, working your rib cage to its full potential means that you are no longer relying on any muscles of the neck and shoulders to compensate for the work your lungs and ribs weren't doing. They can relax and go back to doing their own jobs. Your other "value-added" in this equation is improved circulation, which will manifest as clearer skin, better digestion, and greater freedom from any number of nagging health complaints.

So, how should you breathe? Well, although the rib cage is a cage, it helps to begin thinking of it as more of a go-go cage than a prison cell. In other words, there is a lot of potential for flexibility and movement within it.

Begin by visualizing the rib cage as an accordion. With each inhale, imagine the accordion expanding outward. With each exhalation, imagine it drawing closed.

Now—and here's the really important bit—begin to concentrate on lengthening your exhalation so that it is two to three times longer than your inhalation. Why? Well, it's a common misconception that better breathing begins by drawing in more air. In fact, it begins by more completely exhaling the air that is in your lungs. The more you exhale, the more your body *has* to inhale. While this may seem like a lot to remember at first, it will get easier with practice. The most important point to take away is, no matter, what, keep breathing!

Note: The exercises of Pilates cannot be done with any other breathing than that of the accordion, as you are required to contract your abdominal muscles throughout the work ("scooping") to ensure a strong back and long waist. The diaphragmatic "belly breathing" of yoga and meditation do not apply during Pilates exercises. At no point should you allow the muscles of your abdominals to expand with your breath. This will take practice but is a non-negotiable element in the Pilates system. (I've been told that Joseph Pilates, in his accented English, was fond of commanding his clients to "Pull da stomach in and up!" I execute this "in and up" movement of my abdominals whenever I need a lift in the day.)

the all-powerful powerhouse

Since I'm asking you to begin to work from the inside out, why not take a peek at what's in there? I'm not asking that you be able to identify your muscles and organs by name, as I feel that that has no bearing on what you feel or how you move within your body; this is simply an up-close-and-personal visual reference point for the all-powerful powerhouse. Note the sizes of your powerhouse muscles and the directions in which they run. You can recall this visual knowledge when you are working out so as to get more length from your stretches and deeper contractions out of your strengthening work.

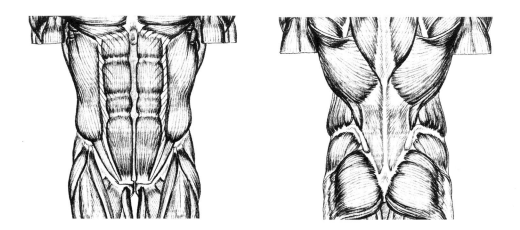

accessing the all-powerful powerhouse

Now that you have a better idea of your own body's quirks and qualities—and you can visualize the location and correct alignment of your skeleton and powerhouse—do the following visualization/exercise to access these critical core muscles:

1. Move to the front edge of your chair and place your feet firmly on the floor beneath you, with the entire sole of the foot pressing evenly into the floorboards and with your heels directly beneath your knees.
2. Pitch your body slightly forward, keeping the spine straight from your hips through the crown of your head, and squeeze buttocks together tightly.
3. Now lift up in your waistline as if being hoisted by wings, separating your ribs from your hips.

4. *Imagine pressing the crown of your head through the ceiling and inserting rulers between your bottom ribs and the top of your hip bones.*

5. With this image of lifting taller firmly in mind pull your belly in and up, as if filling up your back with the muscles from your front.

6. Try to touch your bottom ribs together inside your body without rounding forward in your shoulders.

challenge: Stay in this position and practice your "accordion" breathing without changing one iota of your perfect form.

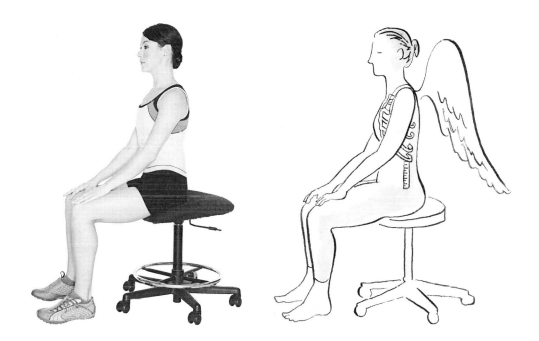

applying the pilates principles to special situations

Every client has days when he or she cancels appointments due to pain, illness, or general malaise. Of course, listening to your body and respecting the messages it is sending you is one of the most important conversations in which you'll ever engage. But what happens when—as can often occur with those around us—you seem to be having the same conversation over and over and there is never any resolution? At that point, my suggestion is to stop and regroup. Is there another way to approach the activity or situation? This section looks at common health complaints and how the application of the Pilates principles might help alleviate or ameliorate ongoing health challenges.

Most of our chronic aches and pains come from poor postural habits. It may sound simple but it's a fact. The imbalances caused from not using our powerhouse, and the ensuing compensation from our surrounding muscles, result in stiff, aching, strained, and pained muscles and joints. We need to begin to think of all of our muscles as a team—no movement taking place without the help of all—and most especially the team captain: the powerhouse.

We need to learn "equal and opposite movements," so we can undo what we've done. To begin, we need to ask ourselves, "What is causing the pain?" Is it from long hours sitting or standing incorrectly at your job? From incorrect workout alignment? From a lumpy mattress? What movements feel good and relieve the pain? What movements don't feel so great? Once you know the probable causes of the pain you can begin to work to correct it.

principles for neck/shoulder pain

There are a number of contributing factors in neck and shoulder pain. Among them, the effects of back muscle tightness that has radiated upward. If this is a common complaint for you, the following principles should provide some relief.

do

- Keep your shoulders rolling down and back, away from your ears, at all times. This will stretch the neck muscles and engage upper and side body muscles.

don't

- Do not try to relieve stiffness by "cracking" your neck or by using jerky movements to "release" tightness.

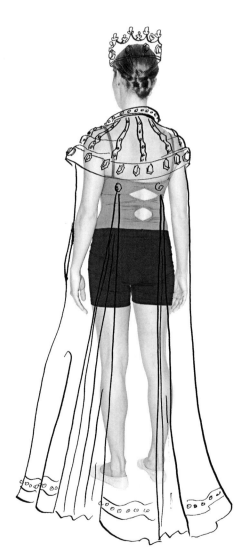

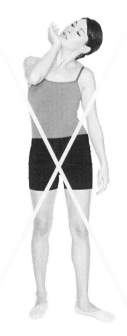

imagine: The weight of a jewel-encrusted royal robe pressing down and pulling back on your shoulders. Press the crown of your head up through the ceiling to lengthen your neck in opposition.

principles for lower back pain

Most chronic low back pain results from poor posture—standing, sitting, and even lying down. One of the first things I look for on a client is whether or not the abdominal muscles and powerhouse are engaged. Engaging these muscles will not only alleviate the pain in the moment but will also isometrically work to strengthen these all-important muscles, contributing to relief from further pain.

do

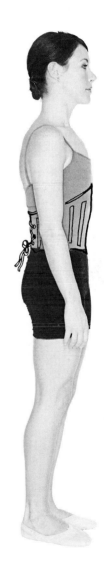

- Stay long in your waist, to avoid crowding or crunching your lower spine.

don't

- Do not lock your knees while standing or exercising, as this puts a lot of pressure on the spinal column.

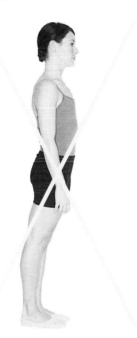

imagine: You have a corset cinched around your waist, lengthening and supporting your back.

principles for knee pain

Most knee pain is the result of poor leg/ankle alignment, and can be alleviated through strengthening the muscles of the hips, thighs, and buttocks.

do

- Keep your knees "soft" (not bent, not locked into extension) to relieve pressure in the joints and engage the muscles of the buttocks.

don't

- Do not roll in or out on your feet. This causes wear and tear on the joint because the majority of the weight rests on only one part of the knee.

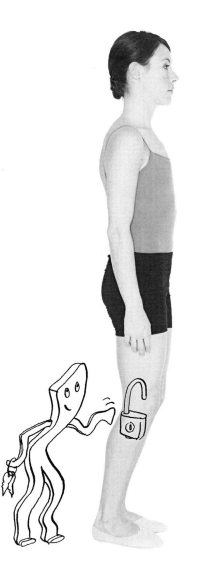

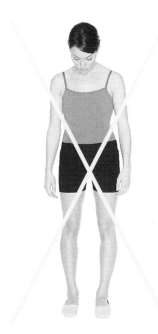

imagine: You are being poked gently behind your knees, reminding you to keep them soft and unlocked at all times. Remember too that all movements of the legs must originate from up in your powerhouse and that the leg is an extension of those muscles.

principles for a sluggish system

There will always be days when you wake up with no get up and go. When this happens to you, the following moves will help you regain the energy needed to embark upon your day.

do

- Gentle contractions of your powerhouse will help with digestion and circulation.

don't

- Don't slouch in your lower back, causing your tummy to pooch and crowding your intestines.

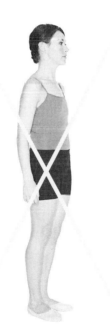

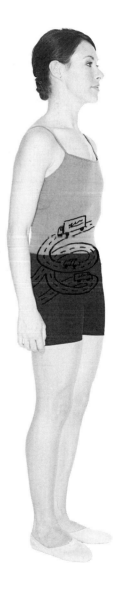

imagine: Your intestines are a highway, through which cars must move freely. Slouching impedes the flow of traffic.

principles for stress reduction

Which came first, the chicken or the egg? Most stress is the result of tight muscles—and tight muscles stress our bodies. Oxygen is a vitally important tool for relaxing muscles and relieving soreness. Remember to focus more on your exhalation than your inhalation.

do

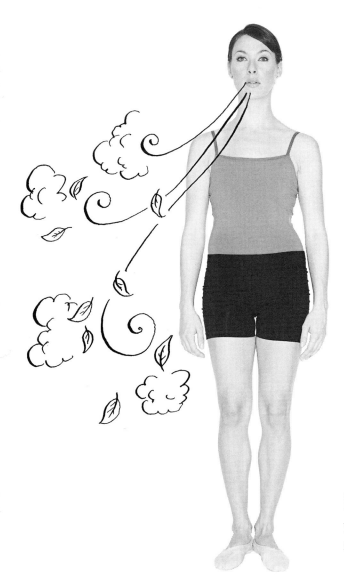

- Make sure you are completely filling and emptying your lungs with each breath. This will help release toxins from your system.

don't

- Don't hold your breath. When you notice you are not breathing, or are breathing erratically, note the area of your body that feels most tense. Then inhale and exhale deeply, concentrating on that spot during your exhalation.

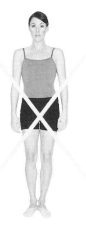

imagine: Being able to blow the stress out of your system, the way a great gust of wind might blow leaves into a flurry of activity.

challenge

Take a look at one of your ongoing health issues. Can you identify the source of your discomfort? Consider your special situation and principles that you can apply to your lifestyle and/or workout so you can still get the benefit of exercise. Is it possible to use some of the modifications introduced here to alleviate your symptoms?

The
Pilates-Conscious
Cardio Circuit:
More Powerful Than Your Pumas, More Necessary Than Your Nikes

"Brooke, no matter what I do, I can't seem to lose these last few pounds." My new client, Sarah, reached a plateau at the gym, and her subsequent frustration has brought her to my studio re:AB®. What can I help her do differently? Just about everything. What will this mean for her? Not only the loss of the last few pounds but less time and energy spent beating herself up—both mentally and physically—on what I've come to think of as the "gym gerbil wheel."

I'm sure I'm not alone in having seen the people whose workouts make us wince—not because of the shape they are in but because they look like they are in so much pain. Or we can tell from their alignment that if they aren't in pain now, they will be when they're finished. You know who I mean: those guys pounding along on their treadmills, taking years off their knee warranties; the women hunched over their stair machines, leaning so heavily on the side handles they might as well be using a walker; the people pumping iron, grunting as they throw around increasingly heavy hand weights, or the girls in sculpt classes watching the clock instead of their instructor. They are there all the time, and they do seem to be working hard. So you're asking "Isn't that a good thing?"

Yes, working hard is good—but working smart is better.

Let's go back to my client Sarah. Her first day, I put her on a treadmill and asked her to show me how she generally worked out. As I suspected, there was pounding, huffing and puffing, torquing and straining. As she continued, I asked her to modify various things: "Lengthen your stride." "Keep your gaze steady." I also asked her to visualize: "Imagine the crown of your head touching the ceiling." Following these visual cues, she was soon moving just as briskly but without making a sound. I could barely hear her steps at all! Meanwhile, sweat was pouring down her face, her alignment was impeccable, and her mind was as engaged as her abdominal muscles. She was working smarter and harder. *Plus,* she was burning more calories per minute—because working more muscles burns more calories. By working from her core, not only was she strengthening her all-important powerhouse, she was burning more fuel in the same amount of time—and you can too.

Interval training—varying intensity during a workout—has long been lauded by the fitness industry for its ability to cut workout time by up to 20 percent, while burning more calories and training the heart more effectively. Why? Because interval training requires that you work aerobically *and* anaerobically. During the aerobic portion of the program your heart is pumping away, using oxygen. During the anaerobic portion of the program you are sprinting, lifting, or jumping—challenging your muscles to go the extra mile and use concentrated bursts of oxygen. Then you go back to aerobic, so your lungs can pay back the "oxygen debt" (the oxygen needed to return to a pre-exercise state).

The upshot? Afterburn, or EPOC (excess postexercise oxygen consumption), which leads to increased calorie expenditure for up to twenty-four hours after you have finished training. In other words, good-bye fat, hello muscle! And don't forget your strengthened heart and capillaries, too . . . which can now more effectively oxygenate your body and flush toxins from your system.

When you move between machines and include weights, bands, and matwork, you create a circuit that will condition your body effectively and efficiently.

The following sections include form notes for using machines, weights and bands, and for developing a personalized mat routine, which you can put together for a total workout whether you are at the gym or at home. Challenges are included, too, to make this book the ultimate full body conditioning tool.

Don't Do Something Else—Just Do What You Do Better! Before we begin walking through the various machines and routines illustrated in *Your Ultimate Pilates Body Challenge,* I would like to take a minute to highlight what is common to them all. You should think of these general form notes as non-negotiable, like gravity. They are a factor in whatever you will be doing, whether you are walking down the street or running on the treadmill. While the non-negotiables may be difficult to put into practice at first, over time they will become second nature.

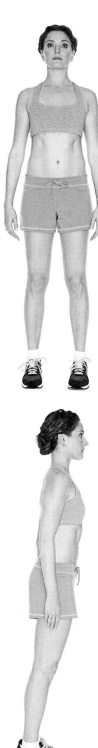

the non-negotiables

Your powerhouse is always engaged: "In and Up." Beginning without this step is like starting to drive without pressing the gas pedal. You might be able to roll along for a while, but you can bet there will be problems down the road.

Your chest is always lifted. Not only is this better for your spine, it's better for your circulatory system, too. If you are hunching, you aren't breathing at capacity. Stand up straight, inhale deeply.

Your spine is a straight line, from its base through the crown. Rounding the back and hunching the shoulders exerts an enormous amount of pressure on your vertebrae. Keeping your spine in a straight line is like taking the kink out of your garden hose: It keeps the energy moving freely through your entire body.

Your gaze is always steady/the crown of your head is always lifted. Not only is this an important component in keeping your spine straight but the mental concentration it necessitates contributes to your workout. As with so many things, where you look is where you go. Looking down will cause your energy to fall. Looking around will lead to scattered thoughts. Watching TV or reading will keep you from engaging with what's going on in your body.

Remember to train your mind to creatively wander through your body as you move, checking in on each area for perfect form and acting as a coach to your team of muscles. Now, with your powerhouse engaged, your chest lifted, your spine straight, and your eyes on the prize, let's hit the gym!

at the gym

Have you ever really watched professional athletes in action? The precision in their form, and concentration in their movements? This control is what separates what they do professionally from what you do in the gym. And why do they work so hard and so well? They have goals in mind—whether adding one more turn to their triple Salkow or shaving a tenth of a second off their hundred meters. They have the desire to win, and they are driven to be the best—even if it's their own personal best. They've also practiced a whole heck of a lot. So I ask you, why not take some of their incentive with you to the gym?

The simplest, most effective workout tip I can offer is to have you compare and contrast your workout form with that of your sport-specific counterpart. Are you someone who gravitates to the treadmill? Channel a world-class runner as you work out. Prefer the stationary bikes? Imagine the superlative form of Lance Armstrong as he cycles to victory. The elliptical? How about taking in the power of a cross-country skier? Observing the techniques of professionals can begin to give you focus and vision. Once your mind can see it, your body can accomplish it!

Having joined my first gym with my dad when I was fifteen, I am certainly no stranger to the evolution of the cardio-machine workout. But it wasn't until my early twenties that I was taught the benefits of proper interval circuit training. My friend, an exercise physiologist, had designed a 1-hour circuit consisting of ten different cardio machines to work all the muscles of the body without exhausting any one group. The concept was a revelation for my body, and my mind! Instead of 60 stultifying minutes on the same machine, of which possibly 20 were performed with proper form, 6 minutes on each machine made the workout much more of a challenge because I then had to make those 6 minutes really count. I began to see the machines in the gym as pieces of a system that, when worked correctly, I could use to change my entire body.

I'd like to change your perception of your gym equipment. This section teaches you how to use your cardio machines in a multipurpose way—so they become a complete workout. Choosing to use more machines for less time, you can begin to build your own circuit at the gym and reap the benefits of interval training. And with all of the technological advances in equipment these days, you can expand the capabilities of your cardio workouts by increasing and decreasing the incline, adding or lessening the resistance, and working to target all of your major muscles in such a way that, on a day when you're fighting the clock, you won't have to hit the weight room, too.

it's not what you do, it's how you do it

Cardio machines are generally of particular use to those looking to lose pounds at a rapid rate or to train for sustained cardiovascular activities (running, cycling, and so forth). However, cardio machines can also add variety to your Pilates workout program and serve as overall maintenance for a fit body. I advocate cardio circuit training in which you work in segments of 10 to 20 minutes on an assortment of machines. For example, a 35-minute cardio circuit workout would look like this: 10 minutes treadmill, 15 minutes elliptical, 10 minutes bike. This interval system keeps the muscles challenged and the mind attentive. Unless training for a sport-specific goal, 20 to 30 minutes of cardio machines followed by a 10-minute mat sequence, three times a week, is perfectly sufficient for body maintenance and will keep you looking and feeling great.

In addition, *Your Ultimate Pilates Body Challenge* provides a 10-minute challenge for each piece of equipment to help turn a seemingly limited stint of cardio into an all-around full-body workout.

When performing the 10-minute challenges remember to work with concentration and control. Find the movements you feel work best and that provide the greatest results for you. Remember too that the ones you hate are probably the ones that are best for you and the ones your body needs. Try creating new challenges for yourself. Always keep your brain inspired, and your body will follow.

T R E A D M I L L S

Few pieces of gym equipment perpetuate the "more is better" misconception than the treadmill. Not long ago I was interviewed for a news story about interval training. The fitness correspondent who interviewed me was an Adonis with bulging biceps and a heaving chest. It was clear he thought the workout he would do with me would be a walk in the park. Laboring under the "more is better" delusion, he proudly boasted that he spent an hour or two a day on the treadmill. I challenged him to do just 10 minutes *correctly*—with his powerhouse engaged and employing visualizations (see right)—and then tell me if he noticed a difference. Needless to say, he was quickly humbled, and I have the videotape to prove it. As with so many things, if you do them correctly, there is no faking it. Now I offer you the same challenge: Forget all that you have previously thought about this machine and envision it as a chance to test your walking and running form and alignment combined with your newfound powerhouse knowledge.

goal: To stay "weightless," so that you barely hear your footsteps as you walk or run—as if you were walking with balloons tied around your ribcage, lifting you.

don't

- Don't fall into your forward-moving foot or let your hip jut out to the side. Stay focused forward and up, *as if balancing a book on your head.*
- Don't roll in or out on your foot. *Imagine creating a balanced imprint with the sole of your sneaker.*
- Don't let your mind wander. Concentrate on achieving your peak performance for a limited time.

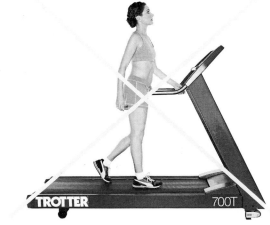

- Stay lifted in your center creating space between your bottom ribs and hips.
- Focus on pressing from your heel through to your toe as you step forward.
- Use the upswing of your arms to help keep your body lifting through space, *as if pushing off ski poles or climbing uphill.*

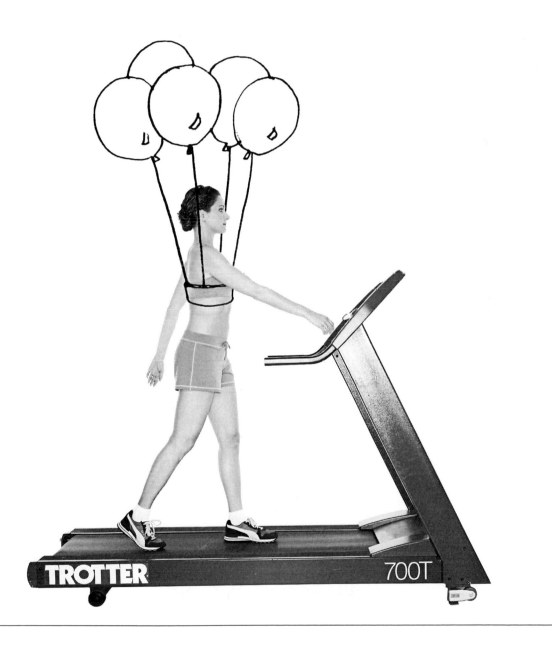

TREADMILLS

TROTTER 700T

10-minute challenge

Every 2 minutes change the dynamic of your walk for a total of 10 minutes:

TREADMILLS

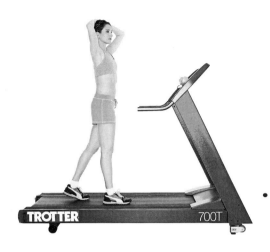

- 2 minutes: Walk with your hands on top of your head (layered one on top of the other, not clasped) (increases your cardio).

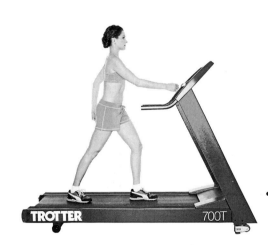

- 2 minutes: Focus on pushing harder with your back foot, as if trying to move the treadmill band without electricity (works your lower body).

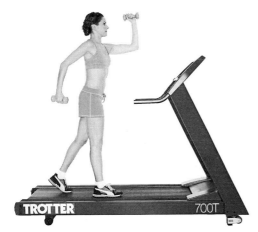

- 2 minutes: Use light weights in each hand (no more than 2 pounds) to increase the pumping of the arms upward (works your arms).

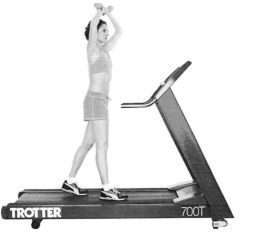

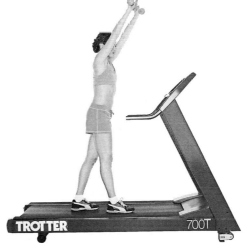

- 2 minutes: Do triceps extensions (bending and straightening the arms overhead) as you walk tall (works your arms).

- 2 minutes: Increase speed or incline without losing form.

ELLIPTICAL MACHINES

Designed to take the pounding off the knees, shins, and hips, elliptical machines often give the illusion that because it doesn't feel like work, you aren't really working out—so you don't have to stay as engaged while you're on them. Not so! When my postpregnant client Debra came in one day and I asked her to start with the elliptical, she said she didn't see the point; she had been on it for 1 hour every morning for the last week, and her last 10 "baby" pounds weren't moving. Wasn't there something "harder" she could do? I challenged her to stay on for 10 minutes, working correctly and following my cues. As her workout progressed, she pronounced, "I never knew it was supposed to feel like this." That's okay, Debra. You're not alone.

goal: To stay lifted and light throughout the workout, as if you were running across a sea of clouds.

don't

- Don't use the frame for support. Use it just to balance.
- Don't let your upper body collapse forward. *Lift your chest as if helium balloons were pulling you upward.*
- Don't read or watch TV. Stay focused on your body.

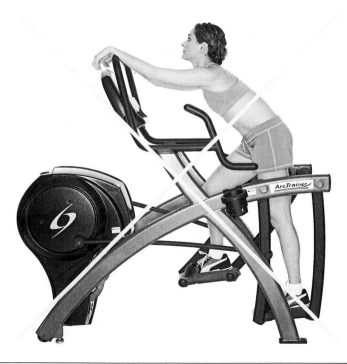

- Draw your powerhouse in and up.
- Keep your entire foot on the pedals, *as if they were stuck with super-strength glue.*
- Focus as much on pulling up as on pushing down.

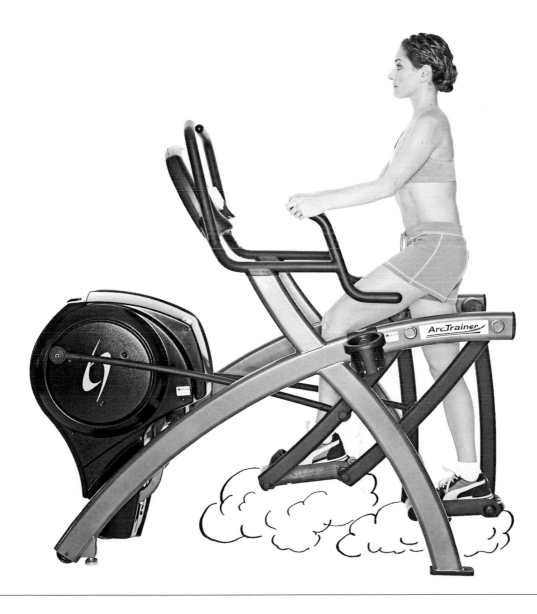

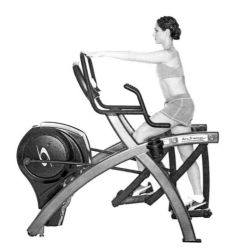

- 2 minutes: Touch the frame with only your fingertips (works your balance).

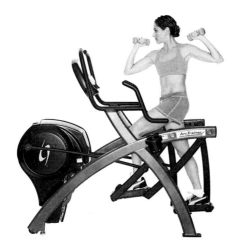
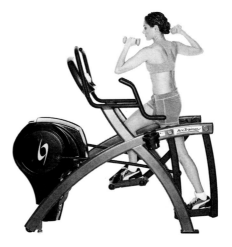

- 2 minutes: Touch shoulders (with or without weights) with hands, lift up and twist slowly from side to side (toward bending leg) with each pedal, working the oblique muscles of your stomach. (Increase elliptical resistance and slow down to do this move.)

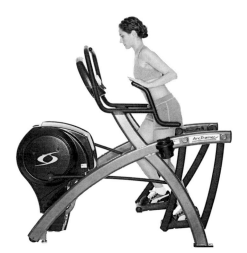

- 2 minutes: Place your hands on the sidebars in a push-up position. Lift the majority of your weight up off the pedals and lengthen your waist—while still pedaling quickly and lightly (works your upper body).

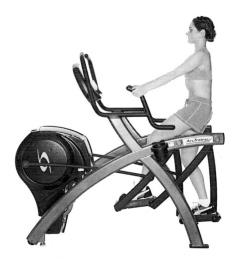

- 2 minutes: Reverse the pedaling direction, soften your knees, and drop your weight into your heels. Try to keep your upper body stabilized—look in a mirror and make sure your head stays in one place (works your lower body).

- 2 minutes: Increase the speed or incline without losing your form.

STATIONARY BIKES

Despite the cliché "It's just like riding a bike!" this happens to be a place I see a lot of people working incorrectly—and consequently getting results that are the exact opposite of what they are striving for. Maybe it's because so many of us grew up freewheeling around on some kind of bike as a kid—whether it was our first tricycle, an old red Schwinn, or our first bike with "racing handles"—we tend to feel like we know what we're doing on a bike. Nevertheless, my client Serena came to me recently and said she didn't want to work on the bike anymore because she felt her thighs were getting too big. I explained that incorrect form was what was making the fronts of her thighs do all the work; I put her back on the bike, had her incorporate all the tips listed below and—voilà!— a full-leg/full-body workout in half her normal workout time. After working correctly, she was showered, dressed, and on her way to a night on the town.

goal: To feel as if you were hovering above the bicycle seat, *as if suspended from a hoist.*

don't

- Don't collapse your shoulders and round your lower back.
- Don't let your knees roll in toward each other; keep them hip-width apart. *Imagine you have a ball between your knees.*
- Don't rock from side to side. Keep your body's weight centered and push from your power-house.

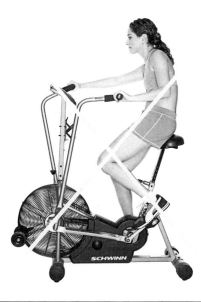

- Stay lifted in your center, *as if you were an hourglass, with a cinched waist.*
- Stay on the balls of your feet.
- Rest your hands lightly on the bars.

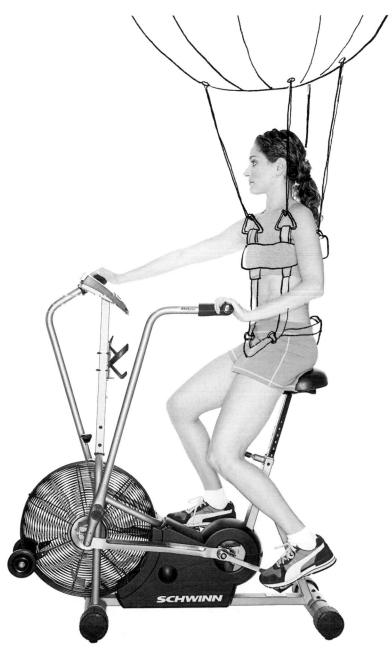

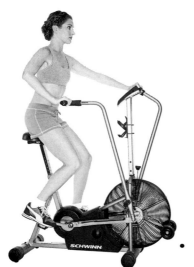

- 2 minutes: *Stick* your feet to the pedals as you pull up (works your lower abdominals).

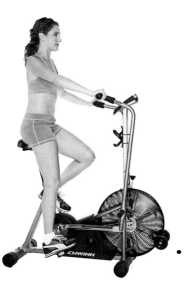

- 2 minutes: Place the arches of your feet on the pedals, and put the emphasis on the down-push (works the backs of your legs).

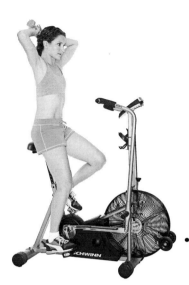

- 2 minutes: Do triceps extensions (see Shaving the Head on page 64) with or without weights; contract your abdominals in and up with each lift (works your abs and arms).

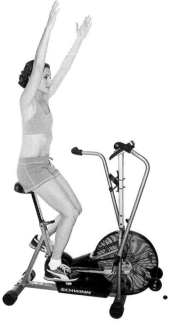

- 2 minutes: Raise your arms above your head in a "victory" pose (increases your cardio).

- 2 minutes: Increase your speed or resistance without losing your form.

STAIR MACHINES

My image of people who have "mastered the stairs" includes many of the ladies from the 1950s films of Ginger Rogers and Fred Astaire: ladies walking beautifully erect up endless flights of stairs, heads lifted, shoulders back . . . gliding like swans. Unfortunately, however, this isn't a visual I often see at the gym. Instead, there are people leaning, panting, and trudging their way "up" with their shoulders shrugged so tightly that they could be earmuffs. The work these people are doing—other than tightening the muscles of their backs and necks—is concentrated in the buttocks and thighs, leading to the kind of complaint I heard recently from my client Rebecca, "My bottom's getting bigger, not smaller!" When she came to train with me at re:AB®, I challenged her to keep her powerhouse engaged throughout—to create the grace and alignment of these early movie stars. Just 20 minutes later, she was dripping with sweat but exhilarated. Her whole body had been worked out, her neck and shoulders were relaxed, and she was ready to tackle her day.

goal: To engage your powerhouse so fully that it looks as if you were being lifted by a pair of angel's wings—gliding, rather than walking, up the stairs.

don't

* Don't let your shoulders ride up around your ears, roll them back and down. *Imagine trying to squeeze a balloon between your shoulder blades.*
* Don't let your bottom stick out. Tuck your tailbone slightly underneath you to take the pressure off your lower back.
* Don't let your feet come off the pedals. Keep them lifting from your powerhouse.

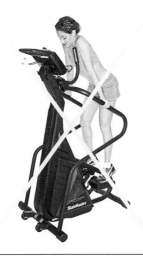

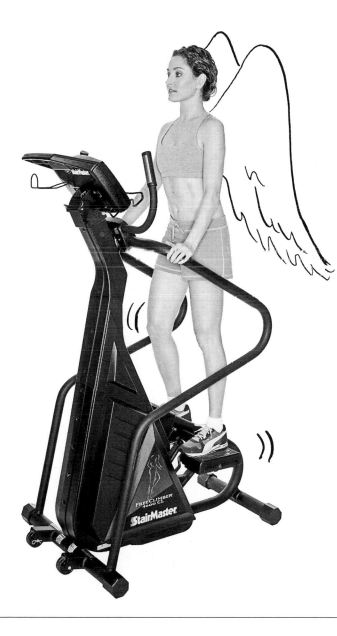

- Keep lifting your chest as you walk or run, *as if you were performing a swan dive off the high board.*
- Concentrate on beginning the lift of your legs from your powerhouse, not your thighs.
- Rest your hands only lightly on the frame.

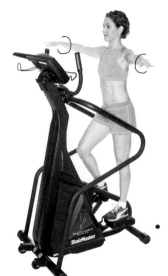

STAIR MACHINES

• 2 minutes: Reach your arms out to the sides circle them outward for 10 circles and then inward for 10 circles, repeating for 2 minutes; make sure you are pulling your shoulders down and together behind you (increases the work in your upper back).

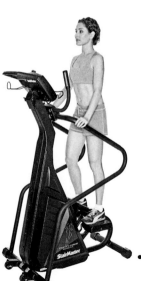

• 2 minutes: Press the pedal with only the weight in the balls of your feet; don't lift your heels up to achieve this—just shift your body's weight toward your toes (works the fronts of your legs).

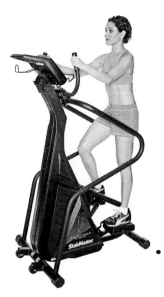

- 2 minutes: Press the pedals from the weight in your heels; don't lift your toes up to achieve this—just shift your body's weight toward your heels (works the backs of your legs).

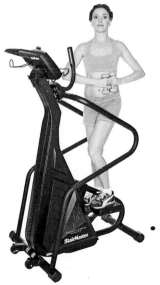

- 2 minutes: With or without weights, lift up and twist slowly from side to side with each step, working the oblique muscles of your stomach; increase the stair resistance and slow down while you do this move (works your powerhouse).

- 2 minutes: Increase your speed or resistance without losing your form.

ROWING MACHINES

This is one place people actually begin by inquiring about correct form. After all, we walk, we run, we climb stairs, but few of us row a boat on a daily basis. Given that, many of my clients don't even want to try the rowing machine. My client Scott is a case in point. Because he is a natural athlete, I thought he'd be thrilled when I first introduced him to interval training on this machine. "No way," he told me, "I'm too uncoordinated." Now, I wasn't going to lie to him. It is tricky to get the timing for the rowing machine in synch. Once you figure it out, however, this piece of equipment is fantastic. Arms, back, abdominals, legs—with your powerhouse in play—you're working them all with every stroke! Joseph Pilates even named a series of exercises after the rowing movements.

goal: To keep a smooth and coordinated rhythm while engaging each and every muscle with every stroke. *Think of yourself as a piece of a larger machine powered by your powerhouse and use the rhythm of your arms and legs to help wind the machinery.*

don't

* Don't let your elbows stick out; keep them close to your sides. *Imagine you're holding hundred-dollar bills under each arm!*
* Don't initiate the movement with your legs alone; pull with your whole body to create resistance. *Imagine pulling stubborn weeds out of the ground using your entire body to wrench them from their holes.*
* Don't let the arm pulley come above the level of the bottom rib as you pull back. It's best to draw a straight line from the wheel to your belly button.

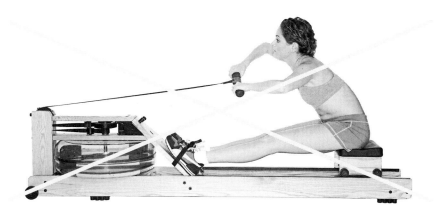

- Get a small to medium-size ball (6 to 8 inches wide) and keep it between your knees when you begin. This will keep your legs hip distance and stop them from rolling in toward one another.
- When extended, keep your legs as straight and strong as tree trunks without locking your knees.
- When rowing back, bring your belly button into your low back, creating a bowl with your belly.
- When rowing forward, stretch long out of your lower back, creating space between your vertebrae. Move with fluidity. *Think of a wave ebbing and flowing.*
- Keep the tension on the arm pulley—both when you pull back and when you are releasing forward.
- Keep tension steady as if pulling the string of a gigantic top.

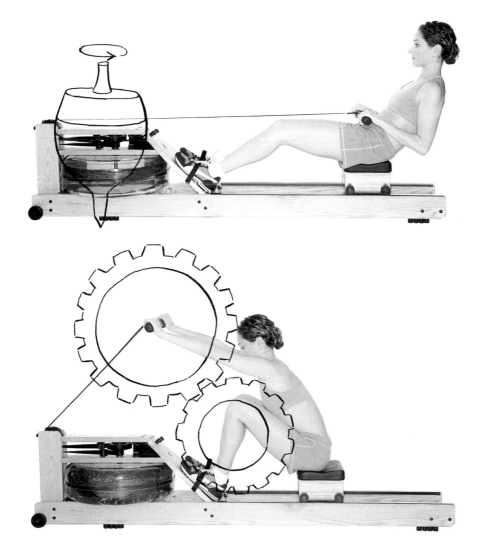

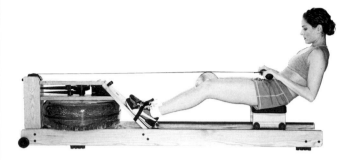

ROWING MACHINES

- 2 minutes: Push through your heels as you squeeze a small ball between your knees (works your buttocks and the backs of your legs).

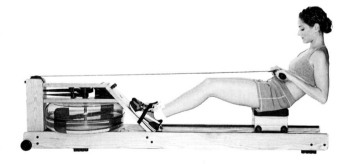

- 2 minutes: Tap your tummy with the bar each time you draw the bar back (works your shoulders and abdominals).

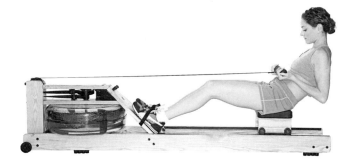

- 2 minutes: Change the position of your hands from palms down to palms up (incorporates different arm muscles).

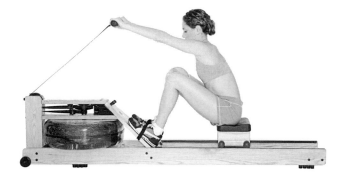

- 2 minutes: Squeeze the ball as tightly as you can while you row (works your inner thighs).

- 2 minutes: Increase the intensity without losing your form.

at home

This section will get you on your way toward realizing the vast number of exercise tools you have at your disposal and how to creatively mold them into challenging routines that break from the norm. Bands and weights don't need to be used every time you work out, but finding ways to incorporate them into your routine can help add variety, challenge, newfound strength, and flexibility.

So many fitness programs today have begun to incorporate bands into their repertoire to help increase strength through resistance, to improve flexibility through a greater supported range of motion, and to work deeper muscle groups. While there is no one established band workout that is universally known and accepted *Your Ultimate Pilates Body Challenge* provides some general form tips you can incorporate into your band work, as well as giving you some new Pilates apparatus–inspired moves to use as interval challenges or on their own.

When you work in interval-challenge style and flow from one movement to the next, you are re-creating the Pilates dynamic used in all the top studios, increasing your aerobic capacity, and burning calories at an increased rate. While slow and steady movement is what I recommend for beginners, when you feel you have mastered the movements to the point of safely being able to move through the ones you know without stopping, you can then begin to challenge your rhythm and dynamic. Up the pace a notch and see how you do. Remember, sweat is your friend! It signals the efficiency of your work and serves to clear your system of toxins and other impurities.

While weights have the stigma of big, bulky muscles attached to them, they are an important part of a well-rounded training practice because using weights helps build and maintain bone density.

Strength training or resistance exercises use your muscular strength to improve muscle mass and strengthen bone. Your muscles are attached to your bones by tendons that tug against the bones when the muscles contract. This tugging stimulates the bones to grow. The stronger your muscles, the more stimulation they provide. The stronger your bones and muscles, the better your protection against osteoporosis.

(ISL Consulting Co. http://health.yahoo.com/health/centers/bone_health/912)

When practicing Pilates in a studio, work on the apparatus can provide approximately 100 pounds of resistance, which serves to increase bone density. For those who don't have the luxury of working in a Pilates studio on a regular basis, free weights can help make up some of the difference. The trick is to work with your weights as if you were on the Pilates apparatus—with smooth, steady, mindful movements. Pilates is a system that is always thinking of the body as a comprehensive whole. As such it is important that a weight routine, normally touted as working segregated body parts, be revised or revamped into a total-body workout tool.

Your Ultimate Pilates Body Challenge provides you with form tips and creative visuals to help put you in the right state of mind to achieve optimum results from modest weight work. In addition, I have provided interval challenges to incorporate your weights into Pilates-Conscious Cardio Circuit routines.

Most at-home routines are fairly lackluster because they are missing concentration and therefore results! When there is no trainer to motivate or fellow exercisers to spur you on it can be very difficult to justify not pausing that video for a phone call or taking a break to throw in a load of laundry. Hence the cobwebs on the weights, the step machine ruining the feng shui under your bed, and the treadmill that has its own dry cleaning license. Again, you're not alone.

So what's so different about what *Your Ultimate Pilates Body Challenge* has to offer? Purpose and focus! When your mind has a goal and your movements have purpose, everything you do becomes more efficient. In this section I give you some general principles you can apply to your daily routine and some sample exercises that you can use to create or add on to your own series.

FREE WEIGHTS

As with the treadmill, free weights are often tools clients use assuming, "How hard can this be? I lift them up, I bring them down." But, as many of you who have spent some time observing your fellow lifters know, the opportunities for incorrect form here are endless.

Joseph Pilates said "Never do 10 pounds of effort for a 5-pound movement." My client Cyril was a case in point. He boasted about doing overhead presses with heavy weights and many repetitions without stopping. As I suspected, he wasn't working with his powerhouse engaged. Instead, he was compensating for the weight and exhaustion factor by throwing his whole body into the lifts, endangering his back with each repetition, and working his periphery instead of his core. I gave him 10-pound weights and asked him to lift them over his head correctly 10 times. It's hard to see a grown man cry.

By now you're probably familiar with the movements of biceps curls and triceps extensions as the staples of a free-weights routine, so I thought we'd diversify and add a few new exercises to your repertoire.

don't

- Don't use momentum to move the weight. Insist on steady, controlled movement throughout; if this means switching to a lighter weight for a while, do so—remember, more isn't better, better is better.
- Don't go limp on the downward motions. Maintain the feeling of resistance throughout; keep the same number of beats for every down motion as every up motion, *as if you are a metronome*.
- Don't lock your elbows or knees.

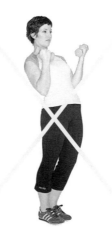

do

- Isolate the muscles you want to work. Give them your complete focus.
- Fuel your movements with your breath. Inhale to begin; exhale to complete.
- Create resistance throughout an entire movement, both as you lift and as you lower.
- Work both arms together. Save single-sided work for strengthening a weaker side.

standing goal: Stabilize your lower body, *as if your legs were the struts of the Golden Gate Bridge,* so that you initiate each controlled movement from your center.

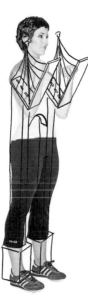

lying goal: Keep your lower back pressing into the bench, *as if you were sewn to it.*

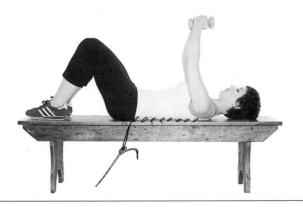

Standing Lateral Raises

1. Take a 2- to 5-pound weight in each hand.
2. Stand with your feet hip-width apart.
3. Engage your powerhouse!
4. Turn your hand slightly at the wrist, so your pinky finger is slightly higher than your thumb. This will engage more of the muscles of the backs of your arms.
5. Lift your arms laterally to shoulder height, at a controlled count of three.
6. Lower your arms to 5 inches from sides of thighs at a count of three. Don't release completely; keep working! *Imagine your arms are wings working against a strong wind.*
7. Repeat 5 to 10 times, with control and concentration.

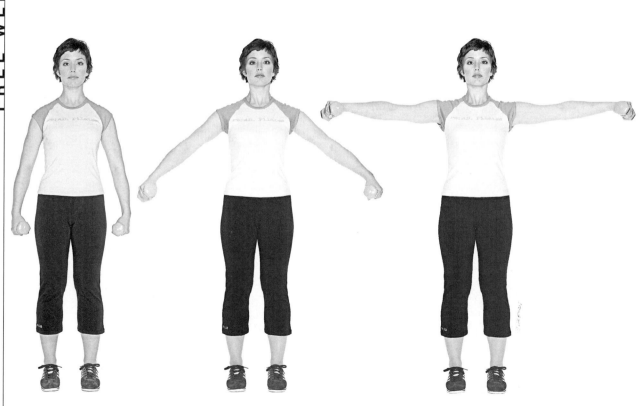

Standing Flys

1. Take a 2- to 5-pound weight in each hand.
2. Stand with your legs hip-width apart.
3. Engage your powerhouse!
4. Bring both hands in front of your thighs.
5. Lift your hands up and together to shoulder height. (Not shown.)
6. Now turn the weights so your thumbs are turned up, and bend your elbows to right angles.
7. Take your arms out to the sides at a count of three.
8. Bring your arms back to center at a count of three. *Imagine you're opening and closing an enormous bellows.*
9. Repeat 5 to 10 times, with concerted effort.

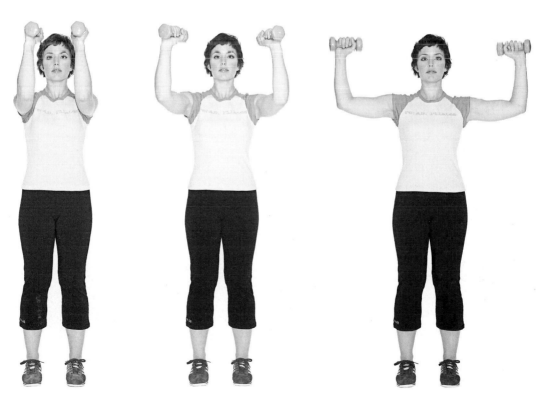

Lying Flys (The Hug)

1. Take a 2- to 5-pound weight in each hand.
2. Lie face up on the bench with your knees bent and feet flat on the bench, hip-width apart.
3. Engage your powerhouse. Don't let your lower back come off the bench at any time during the exercise!
4. Bring the weights up above your chest—not your head—with your arms extended.
5. Turn your knuckles in to face one another and soften your elbows out toward the sides of the room. Keep your shoulder blades drawn down, and your back pressed into the bench throughout.
6. On a controlled count of three, open your arms out to the sides until your elbows are parallel to your shoulders. *Imagine trying to embrace a big balloon as it inflates, then reverse the image and imagine squeezing all the air out of the balloon.*
7. Repeat 5 to 10 times.

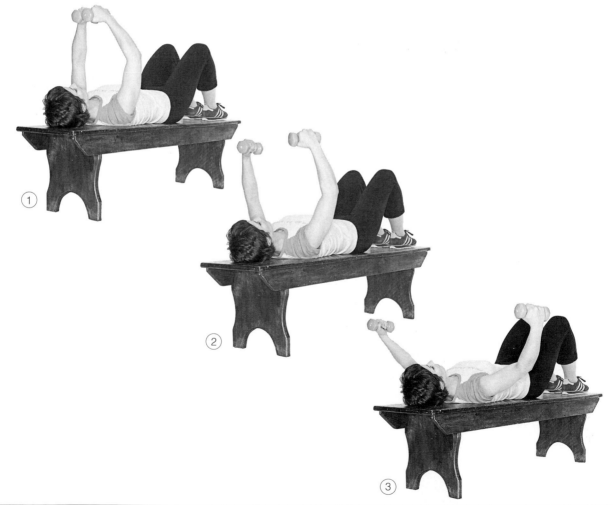

Chest Press

1. Take a 2- to 5-pound weight in each hand.
2. Lie down on the bench with your knees bent and feet flat on the bench, hip-width apart.
3. Engage your powerhouse. Don't let your lower back come off the bench, at any time during the exercise!
4. Bend your elbows to form right angles, with your elbows pointed toward the floor.
5. Using a count of three, press your arms toward the ceiling. Your palms are facing away from you. Allow the ends of the weights to touch each other softly. *Imagine supporting a huge barbell as you reach forward, and then pulling back on two gigantic levers as you bring your arms back in.*
6. Lower your arms on a count of three.
7. Keep your shoulder blades drawn down, your back and pressed into the bench throughout.
8. Repeat 5 to 10 times.

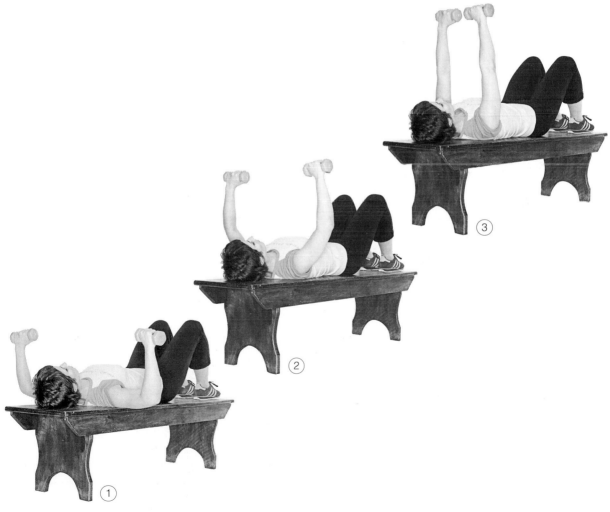

cardio challenge

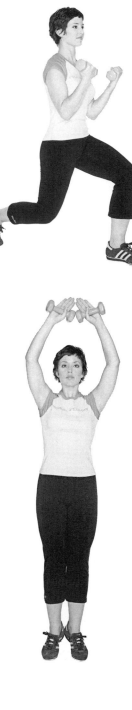

- 10 to 20 reps: Do controlled lunges while simultaneously doing biceps curls (adds work to your cardiovascular system). As you lunge down, inhale and lift the weights up. As you stand, exhale and bring the weights down. Check your alignment carefully. Your ankle and knee should be in a straight line when the leg is bent.

- 15 to 25 reps: Come up on your toes as you do your triceps extensions ("shaving the head") working your calves. (See page 39 for more photos.)

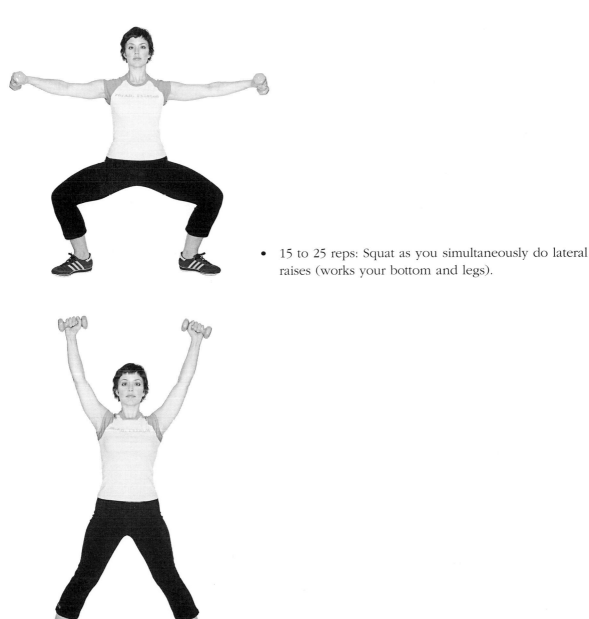

- 15 to 25 reps: Squat as you simultaneously do lateral raises (works your bottom and legs).

- 15 to 25 reps: Slow, controlled jumping jacks (increases your cardio) using light weights only. *To modify:* Bring your arms up only to shoulder height.

- Increase the weight or the controlled repetitions without losing your concentration, resistance, or form.

B A N D S

Bands can often be a mystery. How can something that seems like a toy be so boring to use? Or how can something that seems so easy to use be so unmanageable? My client Elaine found this to be true. She had bought the bands for home and to throw into her suitcase for her frequent business trips. What she'd found, however, was that she was spending too much time using them unimaginatively or—when she did come up with a complicated rigging system—that they had the tendency to throw off her form. The result was that the bands had become one more item gathering dust in her closet, or she packed and unpacked them with feelings of guilt for never having used them. Working together, we came up with a number of Pilates-conscious exercises that maximized both their fun and their effectiveness.

don't

- Don't hold your breath to stretch the band that extra inch.
- Don't initiate from your shoulders. Press your shoulders down and use the muscles along the sides of your body to create stability.
- Don't lock in any of the joints while working with the band.

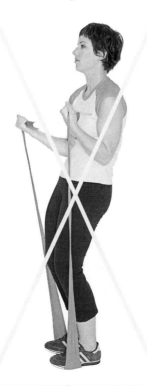

- As you stretch the band, focus on the stable side of your body as well as the side in motion.
- Take as many counts to release the band as you do to stretch it.
- Keep your movements fluid to create rhythm and increase the cardio aspect of these exercises.

goal: To create opposition throughout any given movement, *as if working the plunger of a bicycle pump.*

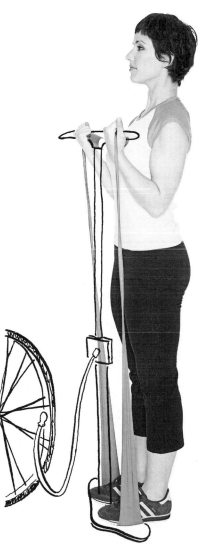

Kneeling Side Bends

Keep a mat under your knees to protect the delicate kneecaps.

1. Place your knees down on one end of your band. Keep your knees parallel about hip-width apart. Leave enough slack in the band to be able to hold the other end of the band by your shoulder. Wrap the extra band around your hand.
2. Inhale, pulling your powerhouse in and up, and stretch the band toward the ceiling.
3. Exhale and bend your body to the side, lengthening your waist while pulling your shoulder away from your ear.
4. Slide the fingers of your opposite hand down your leg toward the floor to increase the stretch, but keep your weight evenly in both knees. *Imagine you are buried in sand up to your waist and unable to shift your weight as you bend to the side.*
5. Inhale and raise your body back to its upright position.
6. Exhale and bend your elbow, bringing your hand back to shoulder height.
7. Repeat 3 to 5 times on each side with concentration and control, deepening your powerhouse with every repetition.

B A N D S

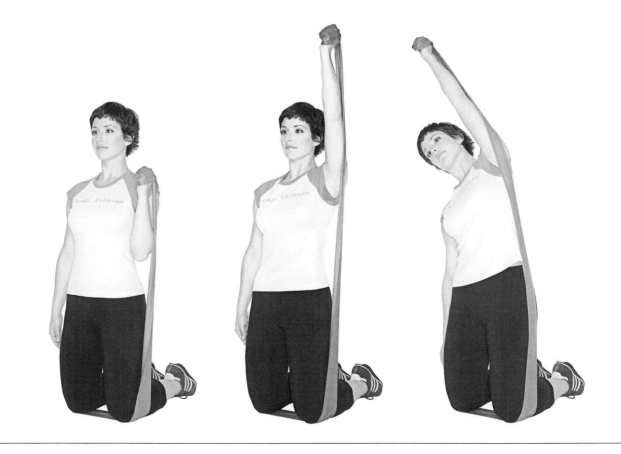

The Frog

1. Lie on your back with your knees bent and open—not wider than shoulder width—and your feet in Pilates stance (heels together, toes apart). Place the band across the soles of your feet.
2. Hold the ends of the bands in your hands with your elbows bent at a right angle and pressed tightly to your sides.
3. Engage your powerhouse and lift your head to look to your tummy.
4. Inhale and press the band away with your feet, pulling your belly in deeper. Don't allow your arms to move.
5. Engage your inner thighs as you straighten your legs. *Imagine trying to stretch out a pair of wet jeans.*
6. Create imagined resistance as you exhale and slowly bend your knees back to their starting position.
7. Repeat 5 to 8 times with concentration and control, deepening your powerhouse with every repetition.

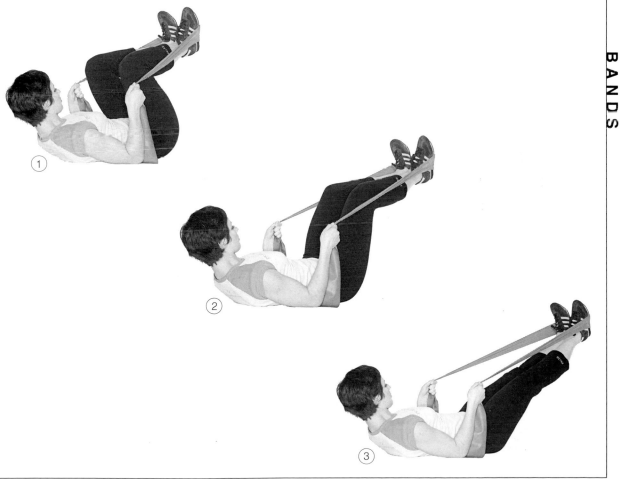

B A N D S

69

Rowing

1. Sit tall with your legs parallel and straight in front of you. Place the band across the soles of your feet while holding the ends in your hands.
2. With knuckles facing each other, inhale as you pull your hands into your chest, sitting taller and lengthening your low back.
3. Exhale as you round your lower back and slowly roll your bottom vertebrae down to the mat one at a time. *Imagine trying to imprint the shape of your spine into wet clay.*
4. Inhale and resist coming up by curling over your own belly to sit tall.
5. Exhale and release the tension on the band.
6. Repeat 5 to 8 times with concentration and control, deepening your powerhouse with every repetition.

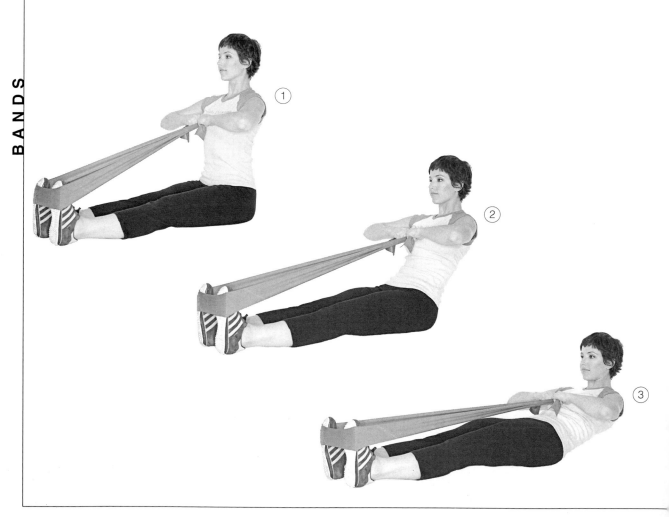

Magic Circle

Use the band like a Pilates magic circle to work your abductors (tie the band into a circle before beginning).

1. Lie on your back with your knees bent and feet flat, about hip-width apart.
2. Make sure your feet are about a beach ball's distance from your bottom. Place the band flat around the outside of your thighs.
3. Inhale to deepen your powerhouse into the mat and pull your knees apart, holding for a count of three.
4. Exhale and try to resist the band's pull as your knees come back together. *Imagine squeezing a big balloon between your knees as you resist bringing them together.*
5. Repeat 5 to 8 times with concentration and control, deepening your powerhouse with every repetition.

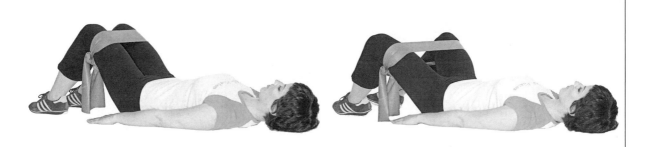

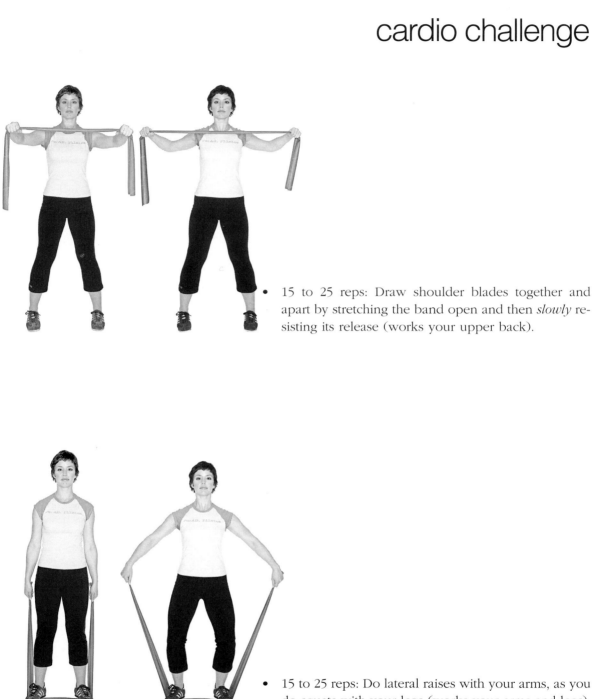

BANDS

- 15 to 25 reps: Draw shoulder blades together and apart by stretching the band open and then *slowly* resisting its release (works your upper back).

- 15 to 25 reps: Do lateral raises with your arms, as you do squats with your legs (works your arms and legs).

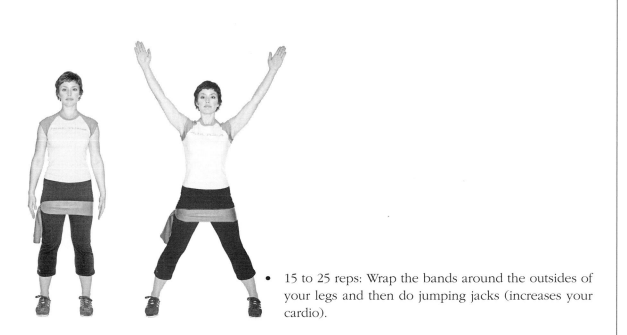

- 15 to 25 reps: Wrap the bands around the outsides of your legs and then do jumping jacks (increases your cardio).

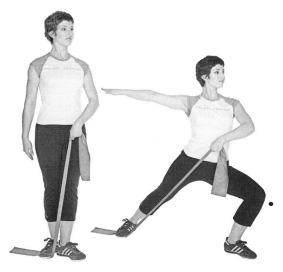

- 15 to 25 reps: Stand on the band with one foot; take your opposite hand and stretch the band as you lunge to the side and twist your upper body to face the lunging knee (works your powerhouse).

- 15 to 25 reps: Increase the rhythm of the movements without losing your concentration or form.

JUMPING ROPE

Many of us had jump ropes as children, and then put them away as "kid's stuff" . . . until we saw a great boxing movie, with a jump-roping sequence that reignited our passion. Having invested in one, however, we discovered that the timing and coordination that had come so naturally on the playground were pretty elusive. My client Dana was anxious to find a fun and easy way to ignite her cardio routine. She'd invested in a jump rope, and then found herself wanting to do anything but jump for joy. Working together, we fine-tuned the form she needed to keep the rope in motion, then added some fancy steps she could use to impress the kids next door.

don't

- Don't arch your lower back. Keep your powerhouse engaged.
- Don't let the movement originate from your legs. Start with your center, *as if propelled by a giant internal spring.*
- Don't hunch your shoulders up by your ears or round them forward.

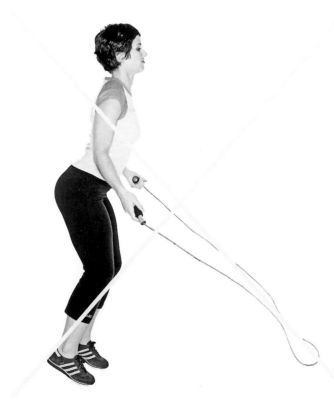

- Keep your knees soft as you land.
- Pick a focal point and keep your gaze there.
- Land as lightly as possible on the balls of your feet.

goal: To keep your landing light, *as if you were jumping on a pillow.*

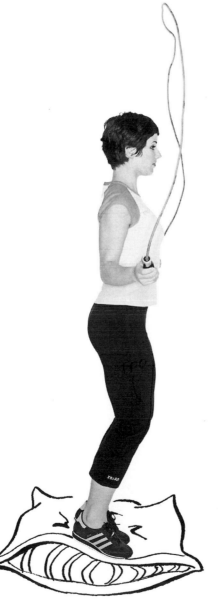

JUMPING ROPE

- 2 minutes: Concentrate on staying in one spot on the floor (increases your focus).

- 2 minutes: Skip forward (increases your cardio).

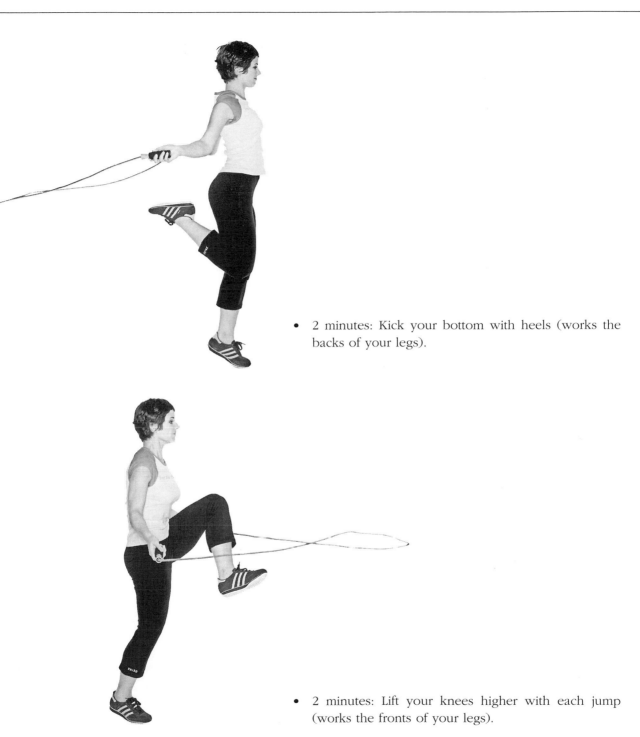

- 2 minutes: Kick your bottom with heels (works the backs of your legs).

- 2 minutes: Lift your knees higher with each jump (works the fronts of your legs).

- 2 minutes: Increase your jumping time or pace, without losing your form.

JUMPING JACKS

Every now and then, I like to have clients do some jumping jacks to up their body's energy. They often remind people of the pure joy of movement they knew as children—when running around was a release and a pleasure, as opposed to a goal or drudgery. Here this old favorite is revitalized into a challenging at-home cardio and strength challenge.

don't

- Don't let the energy of the movement pound you down into your waist or shoulders. *Imagine cinching the corset tighter and lengthening your neck with a high collar.*
- Don't roll outward onto the sides of your ankles.
- Don't let your mind wander.

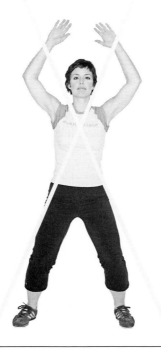

- Stay lifted in your waist throughout the entire jumping jack.
- Focus on squeezing your inner thighs together each time as you bring your legs together, *as if snapping to attention in the army*.
- Use the upswing *and* downswing of your arms to lift you higher in your waist, *as if swimming through the air*.

goal: To keep the energy of the movement up throughout, *as if you were working in zero gravity or in a rocket shooting up off the ground*.

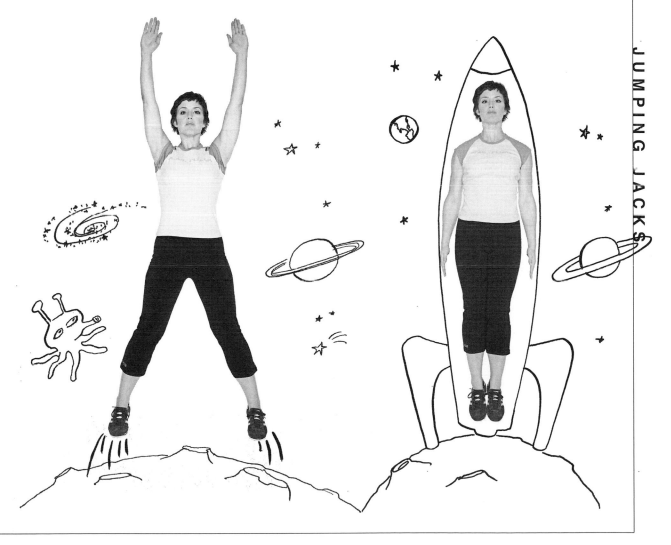

This challenge is only 5 minutes because of its inherent total-body movements.

JUMPING JACKS

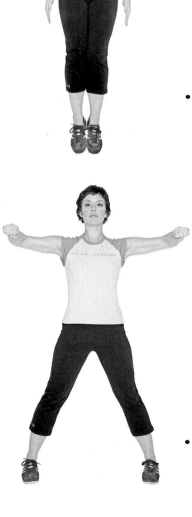

- 1 minute: Change the emphasis of the movement to pulling your legs together and pulling your arms down to your sides (works your inner thighs). *Imagine being pulled into a tight column each time your bring your arms/legs together.*

- 1 minute: Keep your elbows bent, *as if playing an accordion,* each time you jump and jack (works your shoulders and upper arms).

- 1 minute: Change the dynamic to pressing your arms up and pushing your legs apart, *as if doing jumping jacks underwater* (works your hips and outer thighs).

- 1 minute: Each time you land, add a squat, with perfect alignment (when bringing your legs together, squat: feet together, entire sole of the foot on the floor, and knees squeezing together over toes; when moving your legs apart, squat: entire sole of the foot on the floor, and knees open, bending directly over toes) (works your upper legs and buttocks).

- 1 minute: Incorporate as many of the above moves as possible.

on the mat

One of the greatest things about Pilates is that the matwork exercises make your body a portable gym. Much like the Invisible Workout®, the matwork exercises are a way of beating a system that tells you that you must have an expensive gym or trainer to stay fit and healthy. "Physical fitness can be achieved through neither wishful thinking nor outright purchase!" said Joseph Pilates.

I've chosen ten exercises that I consider to be the "meat and potatoes" of *Your Ultimate Pilates Body Challenge,* the Tantalizing Ten is a routine that will be the foundation for the more challenging movements to come. You will find that on its own the Tantalizing Ten will serve you well any day, and everyday; and I ask that you master these exercises to the point of innate understanding before moving forward.

After you're confident with these ten, you will use them as the base for four brand-new routines pulled from various exercises within the mat and apparatus work of Joseph Pilates: Adding Abs, Lean Lower Body, Perfecting Posture, and Finding Flexbility. These four new routines will target your more specific concerns of abdominal strength, toning legs, improving posture, and overall flexibility. Remember that although an individual exercise may target a specific body segment you should always be focused on working as many muscle groups as possible at all times, seeing the body as an integrated whole.

While Joseph Pilates tailored his mat exercises to the individual needs of his students, over the years matwork has been grouped into categories of beginner, intermediate, and advanced exercises to help teachers navigate a safe progression through the system. (In fact, what makes a Pilates exercise "advanced" is not so much the experience or strength of the practitioner performing it as it is the control and precision with which it is consciously performed.

You are the one who must work to find which movements are realistic and best suited to your own body's needs.) To broaden the idea of specific exercise levels I have included Modifications and Progressions to help give you security when you need it as well as the room to grow as you become stronger and more confident.

Why? Because when all is said and done the levels are unimportant to your success. We, in my corner of the Pilates world, affectionately refer to the advanced exercises as the "bells and whistles" of the system. They're fancy and fun to look at but they're not what drives the Pilates method or what makes it so effective. I have created the matwork sequences in *Your Ultimate Pilates Body Challenge* with this in mind.*

As in *The Pilates Body*, I have created progressive mat routines that can be used as your bare minimum for the day or in conjunction with the gym, weights, bands, and sports sections of this book. As you venture into different routines, feel free to mix and match. The only hard and fast rule in Pilates is that you perform every movement with complete control and concentration. Learn one movement well before moving on to the next it is the quality of the movements that will yield the best results. All of the routines that follow have been designed for maximum fluidity from one exercise to the next. You can also slow them down as needed to work on specific areas you feel need your greater attention.

As a general rule, if it doesn't feel good . . . *leave it out!* Do not push through pain in Pilates. Try each exercise and adjust it to your own level by using the Modifications and Progressions until it feels right for your body.

Learn to stay aware of the difference between an exercise that is hard because of the effort it takes (good) and one that is hard because it is painful on your body to execute (bad). When you have found your appropriate individual level of the exercises in question, you will want to work on attaining fluidity and sewing them into a rhythmic routine by way of the transitional moves I provide throughout the matwork sections. These transitions will teach you to tie your movements together into a seamless "dance" that increases your aerobic work. You'll burn more calories and get better stretch from your warm muscles.

If you find certain concepts repetitious, this is no accident. Pilates is really a very simple, and natural, methodology with some complex movements built

*For routines that are broken down into the classic levels, refer to *The Pilates Body* (Broadway Books, 2000).

in. You will notice the following advice and instructions throughout: "tighten your buttocks," "pull your tummy in and up," "press your shoulders down," "squeeze your inner thighs," "lengthen your spine," "cinch your waistline," and so forth. Put all those into practice, and you're practically a master at Pilates already. Now you need to learn to move with all those elements in place and you've got it made!

the rule on "cheating"

I put the word "cheating" in quotes because my idea of cheating may surprise you. If, to give yourself a better stretch to your toes you need to slightly bend your knees while still maintaining good form . . . that's *not* cheating. If you completely throw your form out the window to touch your toes . . . that *is* cheating! The goal of Pilates exercises is ultimately to achieve the widest range of motion possible with the most dynamic flow while still maintaining the integrity of your "perfect" form. You should not expect yourself to be able to do this on your first or fortieth try for all the exercises, although you must continue to push yourself toward your ultimate goal each time. You will find certain exercises at which you are able to succeed wildly and others that need work. That's the joy of this system. It's progressive and goal oriented and should keep you entertained for many years to come. I often say to my Type-A clients who are frustrated that perfection can sometimes elude them, "If you could master Pilates in a weekend think of how bored you would be on Monday."

keeping it cardio

Over the years I've heard a lot of people saying that Pilates is great, but it's "just not aerobic enough." Au contraire. Any authentically trained Pilates instructor—or student trained by such an instructor—will testify that, done correctly, a Pilates workout is an exceptional cardio workout. This myth is particularly disheartening because Joseph Pilates designed his system to combat his asthma by strengthening his lungs and circulatory system; consequently, the best workout to maintain your healthy, cardio-fit body is inherent to the system. The secret is in the emphasis on rhythm and in the use of your "exaggerated" breath—that is, full inhalations and full exhalations. Take any number of matwork exercises and perform them in their appropriate sequence, emphasizing the dynamic and breathing elements, and you've got an aerobic workout to rival the best of them.

pilates stance

In the exercise instructions you will come across the expression "Pilates stance" to describe the stabilizing position of the legs and feet. Pilates stance is a slight turn-out of the legs initiating from the hip joint. Imagine turning your thighs away from each other while your feet remain in a small V position and your heels stay glued together. Your knees should remain "soft" or straight but not locked.

Turning out into Pilates stance by wrapping or squeezing the backs of the upper inner thighs disengages your thigh muscles and engages instead the target areas of the hips, buttocks, and outer and inner thighs.

layering the hands

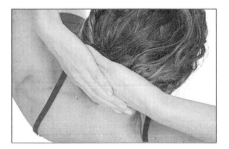

In order to ensure you are working your deepest muscles to lift yourself up—rather than relying on your hands to pull you up—be sure to layer your hands and not interlace your fingers. Try to layer hands palm over back of opposite palm for the deepest work.

supporting the lower back

When performing exercises that involve lowering your legs you may find your back beginning to arch off of the mat—that's a no-no. On the way to perfecting your powerhouse you may find this modification helpful. By placing hands in a small V under your buttocks with thumbs outlining your tailbone, you create a "doorstop" that adds stability to your pelvis and allows your legs to stretch lower. Remember this is an interim measure until you are sufficiently strong enough in your powerhouse to complete the move without help.

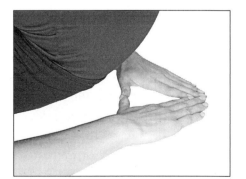

Tantalizing Ten These ten exercises, and one rest position, create an excellent, thorough base routine that can—and should—become second nature to you. This routine can be used as a stand-alone series, or as an accompaniment to a session at the gym or an athletic endeavor.

As you move forward into the subsequent matwork series you will be using these ten exercises as your foundation and inserting new exercises into the sequence. The road maps show you the routine as a whole. I have slotted the new movements into the places I deem appropriate to keep the proper rhythm and flow of the matwork. In Pilates you are never in one position for too long and in keeping with that philosophy and its related cardio results, I have sewn each new series (Adding Abs, Lean Lower Body, Perfecting Posture, Finding Flexibility) into the fabric of the Tantalizing Ten as seamlessly as possible. Instructions on each page will transition you from exercise to exercise.

The routines are not to be combined to form one enormous routine. Meaning, do not add both Adding Abs and Perfecting Posture to the Tantalizing Ten to create an über workout. Instead find what works best for your body, what challenges and changes you, and work the system. You can switch between the routines as often as you like but remember to learn each movement well before progressing or adding on.

While the Tantalizing Ten is the base upon which you will build, each exercise within it is not necessarily basic. To that end I have labeled the levels according to the degree of challenge for a beginner. These levels do not necessarily correspond to previous Pilates manuals as they are not based upon a standard system. The levels are meant to guide those new to these movements so as to remain efficient and, above all else, safe!

The Low Back Stretch at the end of the Tantalizing Ten is for you to use whenever you feel you need to release your lower back or need a break. When used within a matwork routine assume the position for a quick count of three and then move on. If needed, this can be a rest position with which to catch your breath or end the day. Enjoy!

road map

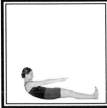

the roll up
beginner

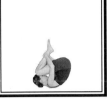

rolling like a ball
beginner

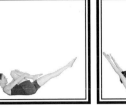

single leg stretch*
beginner

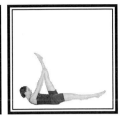

double leg stretch*
intermediate

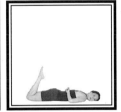

single straight leg*
stretch
intermediate

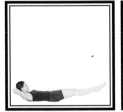

double straight leg*
stretch
advanced

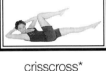

crisscross*
advanced

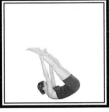

spine stretch
forward
beginner

open leg rocker
intermediate

double leg kicks
advanced

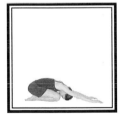

low back stretch

*note: There are five exercises that I call the "Fabulous Five": Single Leg Stretch, Double Leg Stretch, Single Straight Leg Stretch, Double Straight Leg Stretch, and Crisscross. They are a stomach series designed to target all of your abdominal muscles and should be done without stopping or lowering your head in between. Make it your challenge to commit these to memory and perform them every day without fail. You will increase your abdominal strength tenfold!

THE ROLL UP

goal: To create oppositional stretch in your body, *as if resisting the pull of a rope around your lower belly.*

step by step

1. Lie on your mat and stretch your body to its full length, the way you might stretch when you get up in the morning.
2. Squeeze the backs of your inner thighs together, flex your feet into the Pilates stance, and begin to bring your straight arms forward over your head.
3. As your arms pass over your chest, lift your head and inhale as you roll up and forward. *Imagine that your legs are bound together and unable to move as you roll up.*
4. To feel the articulation of your spine, it is helpful to imagine this rhythm: Lift your chin to your chest—lift your chest over your ribs—lift your ribs over your belly—lift your belly over your hips—and *imagine trying to lift up out of your hips and over your thighs.*
5. Exhale as you stretch forward while keeping your navel pulling back into your spine.
6. *Imagine rounding up and forward over a large beach ball to create maximum stretch in your spinal muscles.*
7. Initiate rolling back down by squeezing your buttocks and curling your tailbone underneath you. Inhale as you begin pulling your navel to your spine.
8. Reverse the sequence of the exercise and exhale as you press each vertebra into the mat beneath you. Keep squeezing the backs of your inner thighs together for stability.
9. When the backs of your shoulders touch the mat, lower your head and bring your arms up and over into a full body stretch before beginning the movement again.
10. Repeat 3 to 5 times. End by rolling up to sitting to prepare for Rolling Like a Ball.

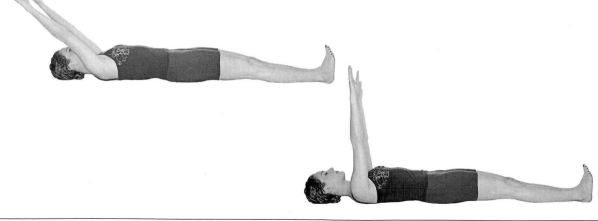

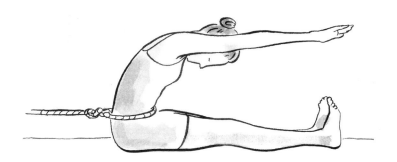

do

- The key to this exercise is to feel the fluidity of movement while not allowing your body to flop forward. This is achieved by using the oppositional force of pulling back in your belly as you stretch forward.
- Remember to squeeze the backs of the inner thighs together to keep the lower body still. *Imagine you are holding a small ball tightly between your ankles or the backs of your inner thighs.*
- Keep your chin reaching toward your chest as you roll up and back down so that you are not pulling from your neck.

don't

- Do not use the momentum from your arms to come up. Instead, use control from the contraction of your powerhouse muscles.
- Do not allow your legs to lift up off the mat as you begin to roll up.
- Do not allow your shoulders to ride up around your ears as you roll up or down.

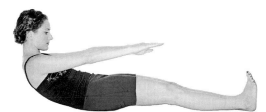

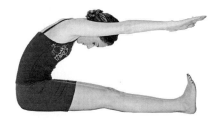

ROLLING LIKE A BALL

goal: To stay tightly tucked throughout the movement.

step by step

1. Sit at the front of your mat with your knees bent into your chest and open slightly.
2. Grab your ankles and lift your feet off the mat until you are balancing on your tailbone. Tuck your chin into your chest.
3. Initiate the rolling by sinking your navel deep into your spine and leaning backward, bringing your knees with you. Do not throw your head back to begin the movement, work instead from your abdominal muscles.
4. Inhale as you roll back to your shoulder blades, and exhale as you come forward, placing emphasis on pulling your heels in tightly to your buttocks as you come up. Work from your abdominals and not your shoulders.
5. *Imagine you are tucked up inside a soap bubble and trying not to pop it.*
6. Each time you come forward "put on the brakes" by pulling your tummy in opposition to your thighs, and balance on your tailbone. Do not allow your feet to touch the mat.
7. Repeat 8 to 10 times. End by putting the soles of your feet on the mat and lifting your bottom back and away from your heels to prepare for the Single Leg Stretch.

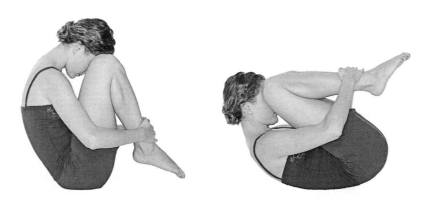

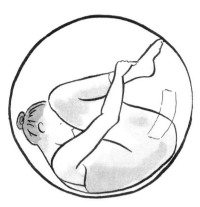

do

- Momentum is the key here. The more slowly you roll back, the less chance you have of making it back up to a sitting position.
- As you roll backward and forward try to feel each vertebra touch down in ascending and descending order *like keys on a xylophone.*

don't

- Make sure you do not allow your head to fly back and forth throughout the movement. Keep your chin securely tucked.
- Do not allow your shoulders to creep up around your ears.
- Do not roll back onto your neck: Stop at the shoulder blades instead.

modification: If this movement is too difficult in the beginning, try placing your palms on the underside of your thighs. Remember to *pull in* your abdominals and to keep your head and neck supported throughout the rolling movement.

progression: For an added challenge try wrapping your arms around your knees instead of holding at the ankles.

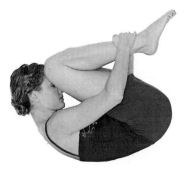 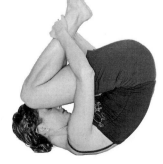

SINGLE LEG STRETCH

goal: To extend your reaching leg in opposition to your powerhouse while remaining still in your upper body.

step by step

1. Sitting with your knees bent, take hold of your right leg and pull it into your chest with your inside hand on the knee and your outside hand on the ankle. (This will keep your leg in the proper alignment with your body.)
2. Roll your back down to the mat bringing your bent leg with you.
3. Extend your opposite leg out in front of you and hold it above the mat at an angle that allows your back to remain flat on the mat.
4. With your elbows extended and your chin lifted onto your chest, inhale and sink your navel deep into your spine.
5. Exhale and switch legs, bringing the outside hand to the ankle and the inside hand to the knee. Stretch your extended leg long out of your hip and in line with the center of your body.
6. *Imagine you are using your extended foot to give a push to a child on a swing.*
7. Repeat 5 to 10 sets. End by pulling both knees into your chest to prepare for the Double Leg Stretch.

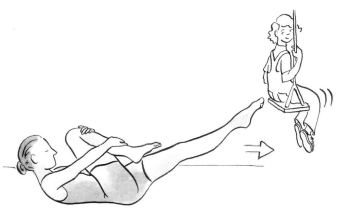

do

- Remember to stay lifted from the abdominals and the back of the chest region and not from the neck itself. (If your neck gets tired, rest your head down on the mat and then try again to lift correctly.)
- Squeezing the buttocks as you extend your leg will help ensure the integrity of the position.
- Keep your elbows extended and your shoulders pressing down and away from your ears to best use your abdominals.

don't

- Don't let your extended leg fall below hip level. Keep the extended leg at a height that enables you to maintain a flat back.
- Don't let your powerhouse disengage as you switch legs. Scoop your belly in at all times and press your spine further into the mat as you switch.

modifications: If you have a bad knee, pull your leg in from the underside of the thigh instead of from the top of the knee. (Do not grab behind the actual knee, as it is a very sensitive area and will most likely prove to be uncomfortable.) For a bad back, extend the straight leg to the ceiling only. As your lower abdominal strength improves, you will be able to begin lowering the leg to a more challenging angle.

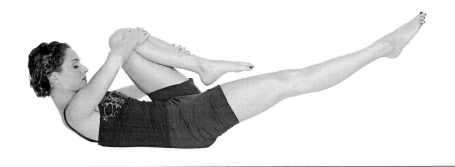

DOUBLE LEG STRETCH

goal: To remain perfectly still in your center, chin into chest, throughout the movements.

step by step

1. Lie on your back with both knees pulled into your chest, elbows extended and head lifted.
2. Inhale deeply and stretch your body long, reaching your arms back over your head, and your legs long out in front of you and raised off the mat about 45 degrees.
3. As you exhale, draw your knees back into your chest and circle your arms around to meet them.
4. *Imagine you are backstroking through peanut butter.*
5. Pull your knees deeply into your chest to increase the emphasis on the exhalation, *as if you were squeezing the air out of your lungs.*
6. Repeat the sequence 5 to 10 times, remaining still in your torso as you inhale to stretch and exhale to pull. End by pulling both knees into your chest with a deep exhalation and go on to the Single Straight Leg Stretch.

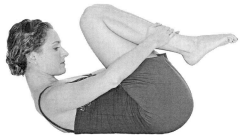

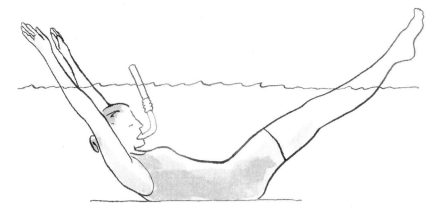

do

- Pull your chest up to your knees as you exhale and keep your elbows extended to feel a nice release stretch in the trapezius region (upper back and neck area).
- As you inhale and stretch out, make sure your arms are straight and you are reaching in opposition to your legs.
- Squeeze your buttocks and inner thighs together tightly as you extend your legs to support your lower back.

don't

- Do not let your head fall back as you stretch your arms above your head! Keep the neck supported by staying completely still in the upper body as you perform the movement (chin to chest).

modifications: For a sensitive lower back, straighten your legs to the ceiling instead of to 45 degrees. As your lower abdominal strength increases, you will be able to begin lowering the legs to a more challenging angle. For a bad neck; leave this exercise out until you feel you have the abdominal strength to lift and support your head and neck correctly.

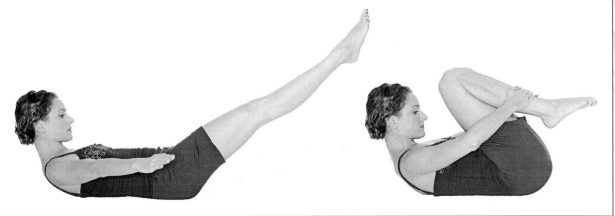

SINGLE STRAIGHT LEG STRETCH

goal: To pull from the ankle without rocking in your upper body.

step by step

1. Lie on your back. Extend your right leg straight up to the ceiling and grab the calf, or ankle if possible, with both hands as you stretch the left leg long in front of you, keeping it hovering slightly above the mat.
2. Anchor your torso firmly to the mat and lift your head onto your chest. Make sure you feel your spine pressing down into the mat beneath you.
3. While remaining absolutely still in your torso, pull the raised leg in toward your head (keeping it straight). Quickly switch the straight legs by scissoring them past each other.
4. *Imagine your legs are as straight and strong as those of a soldier marching in combat boots.*
5. Repeat the motion, inhaling for 1 set and then exhaling for 1 set.
6. Complete 5 to 10 sets. End by bringing both legs together at a 90-degree angle in the Pilates stance, and place your hands behind your lifted head to prepare for the Double Straight Leg Stretch.

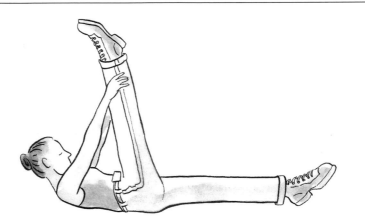

do

- Use rhythm to control the dynamic of this exercise with small pulses on each stretch.
- Keep your eyes focused on your belly and make sure that it is scooping at all times. Do *not* rely on your shoulders to hold the weight of your leg overhead, use that powerhouse!

don't

- Don't let your upper body move when transitioning from the previous exercise.
- Don't sink into your shoulders. Keep lifted from the back of the chest area instead.

modification: If this stretch proves too difficult in the beginning, hold lower down on the leg. Try the calf first, and if it is still too difficult, move your hands to the back of the thighs. Do *not* hold behind the knee.

progression: For a more advanced version, try the exercise with your arms long by your sides. Use control and common sense. If it hurts your neck or lower back . . . STOP!

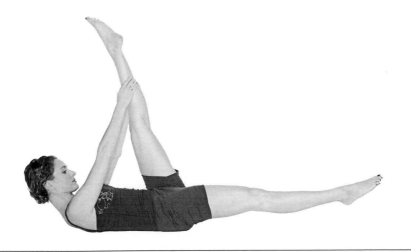

DOUBLE STRAIGHT LEG STRETCH

goal: To keep your center glued to the mat and remain still in your upper body.

step by step

1. Lie on your back with your hands, one on top of the other and *not* interlaced, behind your lifted head, your legs extended straight to the ceiling in the Pilates stance. Squeeze your inner thighs together until no light comes through them.

2. Make sure your torso is anchored flat to the mat and your head is lifted onto your chest without overstretching the muscles in the back of the neck. Do not allow your hands to pull the weight of your head forward. Use your abdominals and upper back muscles to lift you.

3. Squeeze your buttocks, for stability in the lower back, and begin lowering your straight legs down toward the mat as you inhale. STOP if you feel your lower back arch off the mat.

4. Squeeze your buttocks tighter and exhale as you raise your straight legs toward the ceiling. Feel your chest pressing slightly toward the legs as they return to their upright position. *Imagine you have a bowling ball on your powerhouse, pinning it to the mat.*

5. Focus on keeping the head and torso (remember that includes the hips!) absolutely still as you lower and raise the legs. It will help if you do not allow your legs or feet to pass your belt line. Stop them when they are directly perpendicular to the ceiling.

6. Repeat 5 to 10 times. End by bringing both knees into the chest to prepare for the Crisscross.

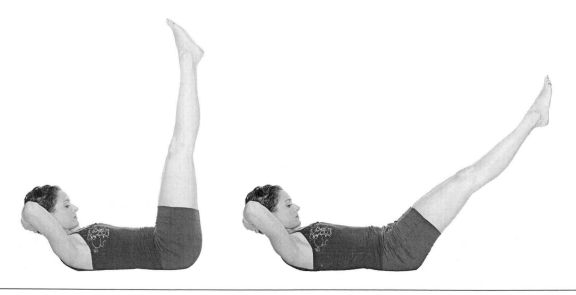

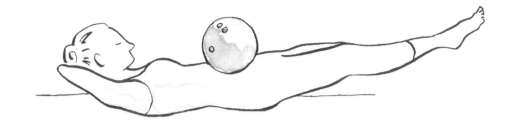

do

- In the beginning, and for as long as it serves you, try tucking your hands in a triangle just below your tailbone (palms down). This position will help support the lower back as it slightly tips your pelvis back toward your center.
- Make sure to keep your elbows out wide and press your shoulders down and away from your ears to stretch the muscles of the neck and further increase the focus on the abdominals.
- To accentuate the control element of this movement, keep a slight turn out in your thighs and squeeze them tightly as you bring your legs back up, pressing your chest toward your thighs as you do.

don't

- Do not lower your legs past the point of comfort for your spine. Make sure you maintain a scoop in your belly throughout the movement, and keep your back pressing into the mat.

progression: For an added challenge, try changing the dynamic of the exercise by switching the accent from the lifting *up* to the lowering *down*. (Change the breath accordingly.)

CRISSCROSS

goal: To keep your center rooted to the mat while twisting.

step by step

1. Lie on your back with your hands behind your lifted head and shoulders, and your knees bent into your chest.
2. Extend your left leg out long—about 6 inches off the mat—while twisting your upper body until your left elbow touches your right knee. Inhale as you lift.
3. Look back to your left elbow to increase the stretch and hold the position as you exhale. Make sure your upper back and shoulders do not touch the mat as you twist and hold the stretch.
4. Switch the position by inhaling and bringing your left elbow to your right knee while extending the opposite leg out in front of you. Hold the stretch as you exhale completely.
5. *Imagine you are pinned to the mat by an anchor, so that you can't rock from hip to hip.*
6. Complete 5 to 10 sets and then pull your knees into your chest.
7. Roll up to sitting and straighten your legs out in front of you to prepare for the Spine Stretch Forward.

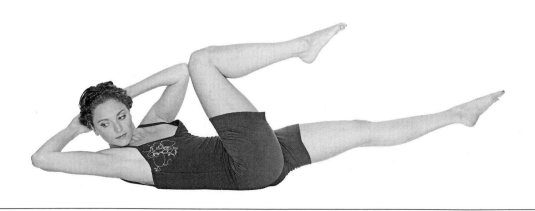

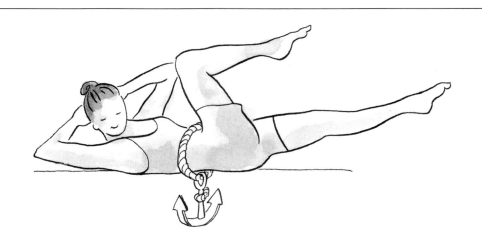

do

- Make sure you are lifting from below your shoulder to reach the knee and not simply twisting from the shoulder socket.
- Keep your elbows extended as much as possible throughout the movements. Do not allow them to fold in or to touch the mat as you twist.
- Be sure to actually look back to your elbow as you twist so you can work deeper into your obliques and even strengthen your ocular (eye) muscles!

don't

- Do not rush through this exercise. Really feel the twist and hold the position as you exhale completely.
- Do not allow your outstretched leg to drop too low in front of you. Maintain control by squeezing the buttock.
- Do not rock your body from side to side. The steadier you remain, the more efficiently you work!

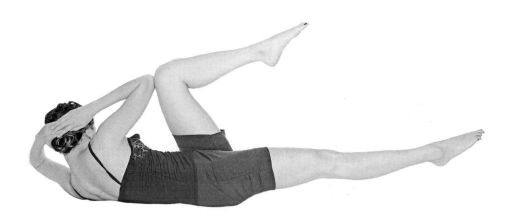

SPINE STRETCH
FORWARD

goal: To increase the stretch down your spine with each repetition.

step by step

1. Sit up tall with your legs extended straight out on the mat and open to shoulder-width.
2. Extend your arms straight out in front of you and flex your feet, *as if you were pressing your heels into the wall across the room.*
3. Initiate the Spine Stretch Forward by inhaling and pulling your navel deeply up your spine. At the same time, sit up even taller by *imagining the crown of your head pressing up and through the ceiling above.*
4. Bring your chin to your chest and begin to round forward.
5. *Imagine you can articulate the vertebrae of your spine like a bendy straw.*
6. Exhale as you stretch forward, being careful not to roll forward from your hips. This is opposition at work again. Your pelvis should remain still at all times.
7. Begin to inhale and reverse the motion of the exercise.
8. Exhale as you return to your tall seated position. Press your shoulders down.
8. Repeat 3 times. End by sitting tall and bending your knees toward chest to prepare for the Open Leg Rocker.

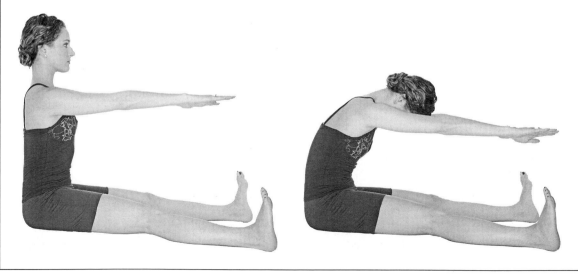

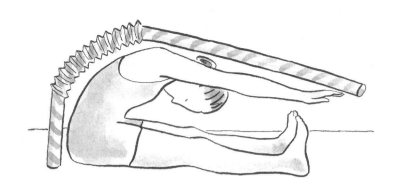

do

- If the stretch in your hamstrings (underside of the legs) proves too much, simply "soften" your knees to relieve the tension. As you progress, try to increase that stretch by straightening one leg and then the other as you exhale forward.
- As you roll up to sitting, make sure you are lifting from your powerhouse to initiate the movement. Your head should be the last piece to come up.
- Press your shoulders down and away from your ears as you roll yourself back up to release the muscles in the back of the neck.

don't

- Don't let your knees roll in as you stretch forward. Think of pulling your toes toward you.
- Remember not to sit back but up as you go.

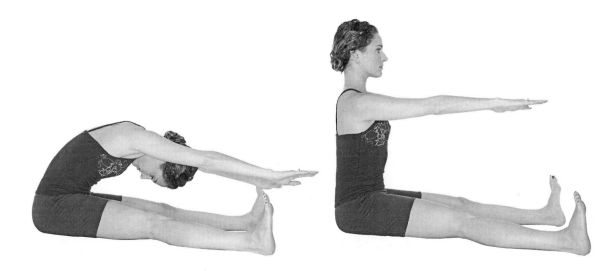

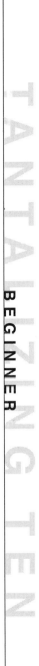

OPEN LEG ROCKER

goal: To be able to rock with straight legs and straight arms, using your powerhouse.

step by step

1. Sit in the middle of your mat with your knees bent in toward your chest. Open your knees to shoulder-width apart and take hold of your ankles (thumbs on top). Pull your navel deep into your spine, and lean back until you are balancing on your tailbone with your feet off the floor.

2. Begin straightening both legs toward the ceiling in an open V position and balance. Your arms are straight. (You can hold backs of calves if necessary.)

3. To initiate the rocking, inhale, pressing your navel down into your spine, and bring your chin to your chest. Do not initiate the movement by throwing your head back.

4. Roll back just as far as the bottom of your shoulder blades, remaining in your V position, and then exhale to come back up.

5. *Imagine being weighted like a punching clown or bottom-heavy piece of fruit.*

6. Repeat 3 to 5 times. End by coming up and balancing to prepare for the Double Leg Kicks.

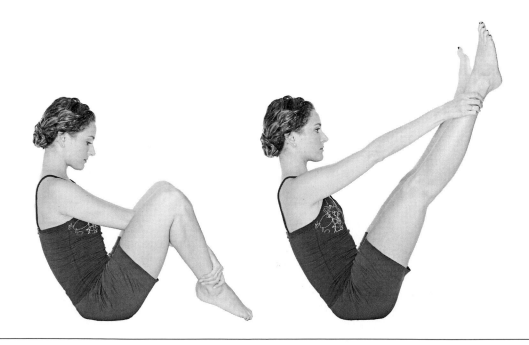

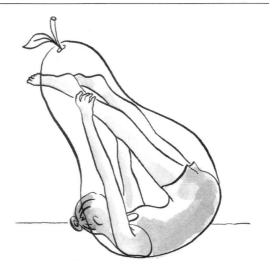

do

- Keep your legs and arms as straight as possible throughout the rocking sequence.
- Work from your abdominals to keep from straining as you come up. Dynamic is the key.
- Roll to shoulders in the beginning and to the bottom of your shoulder blades as you progress.

don't

- Don't roll back onto your neck! Use your abdominals to control the range of movement.
- Do not pump your legs to create momentum.

progression: For an advanced challenge, rock without holding on. Remember to initiate from the powerhouse! Hold arms forward and balance at the top of each rocker.

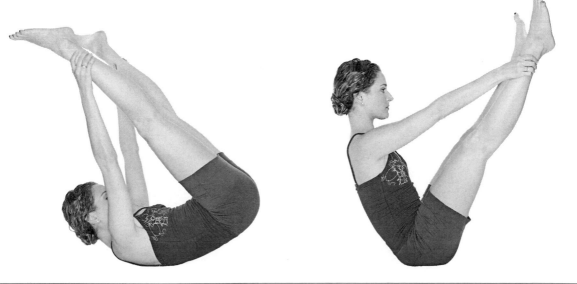

DOUBLE LEG KICKS

goal: To touch your heels to your buttocks during the kicks; to press your elbows into the mat with your hands high on your back; to keep your legs together and your feet down when stretching your back.

step by step

1. Lying on your stomach with your face resting on one side, clasp your hands behind you and place them as high up on the back as is comfortable while still being able to touch the fronts of your shoulders and elbows down to the mat.
2. Squeeze your buttocks and inner thighs together and exhale as you kick both heels to your bottom, *as if you had a fish's tail*, 3 times.
3. As you extend your legs to the mat, inhale and stretch your arms back to follow them. Bring your chest off the mat and stretch your head forward.
4. Continue to reach your clasped hands long and low behind you, squeezing your shoulder blades together and lengthening your spine.
5. Keep your legs and the tops of your feet pressing down into the mat as you stretch back to them.
6. Exhale as you return your upper body to the mat, turning your face to the other side and bringing your hands and heels back to the initial kicking position. Remember to make sure that your shoulders and elbows are able to touch the mat with your hands clasped high up on your back.
7. *Imagine your hands and feet are connected by a spring.*
8. Complete 3 sets.

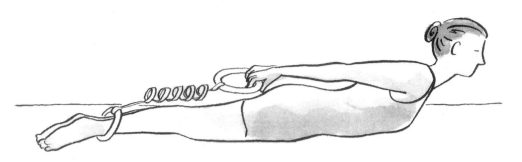

do

- Make sure to keep the arms reaching long and low behind you. Think of trying to get them down past your buttocks.
- Try to keep the tops of your feet pressing into the mat as you stretch back, engaging the muscles of the buttocks and thighs throughout.
- Make sure you are pulling your navel up into your spine throughout to support your lower back.
- If you feel pain in your back . . . STOP! Sit into the Low Back Stretch position.

don't

- Do not allow your buttocks to lift up as you kick your heels to them.

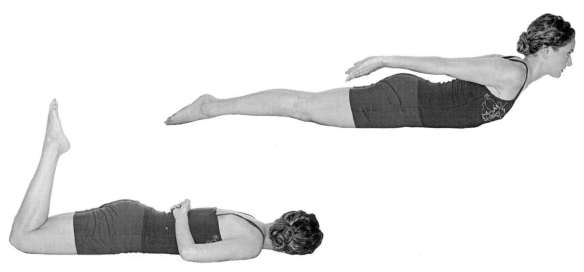

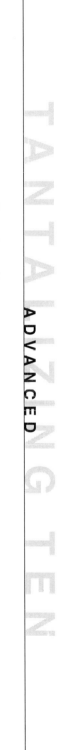

LOW BACK STRETCH

goal: To keep pulling your powerhouse away from your thighs.

step by step

While not an official exercise, this position allows the muscles of your back to stretch from the extension position that precedes it. When performing this stretch in the middle of a series do not linger for more than a moment or you will break your flow. You can also use this position to rest your back at the end of a series if you feel any tension has accumulated there.

1. Kneel on your mat, and then sit your buttocks to your heels.
2. Bow forward and place your forehead on the mat.
3. Reach your arms forward and away from your waist.
4. Make sure to keep your bottom as close to your heels as possible without collapsing, *as if gently resisting the weight of a child sitting on your lower back.*
5. Continue to pull your tummy up into your spine and away from your thighs to increase the stretch of your back muscles.
6. When transitioning to the next exercise, inhale and engage your powerhouse muscles as you roll up to a seated position with your bottom on your heels. Your head should be the last piece to come up.

modification: If you have bad knees, leave this position out. Instead, lie on your back and gently pull the backs of your thighs in toward your chest to release your lower back muscles.

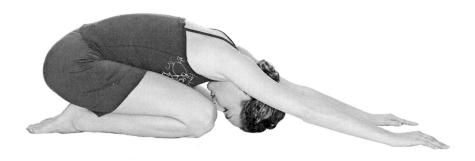

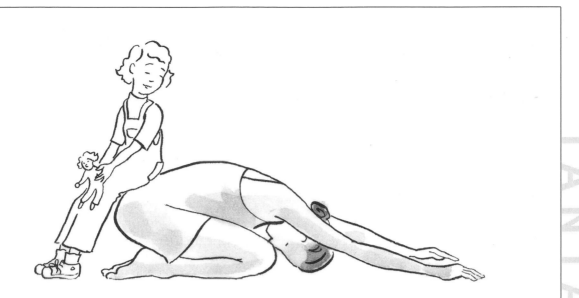

Adding Abs Pilates is a system based around the abdominal region, and every single exercise should initiate and emanate from these stabilizing muscles. This can be easier said than done. Good news! Even before you have mastered the ability to keep your abdominals as the primary focus of all the movements, some Pilates exercises are more inherently prone or geared to be felt strongly in the abdominals (picture the classic sit-up, when done any which way, it must still be felt in the abdominals). The Adding Abs series is designed to target your abs without question. This said, remember not to forget about the rest of your body. The better able you are to maintain correct form (with many muscles of the body engaged), the deeper you will feel the work in the correct place. Remember that the indicated levels are merely guides and you should use the Modifications, Progressions, and your own intuition to help you find your perfect level.

note: The Tantalizing Ten exercises are shown on the road map to indicate their placement within the new series. The instructions in the following pages pertain to the new Adding Abs exercises. I have slotted the new movements into the places I deem appropriate to keep the proper rhythm and flow of the matwork. In Pilates you are never in one position for too long and, in keeping with that philosophy and its related cardio results, I have sewn each new exercise into the fabric of the Tantalizing Ten as seamlessly as possible. Instructions on each page will transition you to and from exercise to exercise. Remember to stay focused on your goal of increasing the strength of your abdominals throughout the execution of each movement without neglecting the other muscles of your body. Your entire body is working toward the goal of a firm midsection.

road map

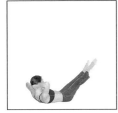

footwork
intermediate

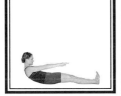

roll up
beginner

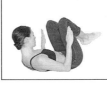

stomach massage I
advanced

coordination
advanced

rolling like a ball
beginner

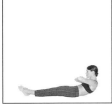

rowing I
advanced

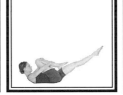

single leg stretch
beginner

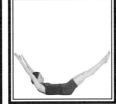

double leg stretch
intermediate

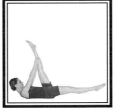

**single straight
leg stretch**
intermediate

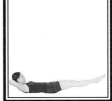

**double straight
leg stretch**
advanced

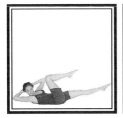

crisscross
advanced

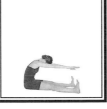

**spine stretch
forward**
beginner

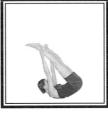

open leg rocker
intermediate

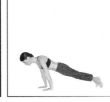

long stretch
intermediate

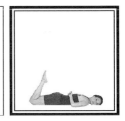

double leg kick
advanced

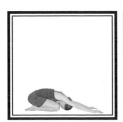

low back stretch

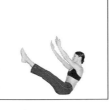

reformer teaser
intermediate

F O O T W O R K

goal: To deepen the powerhouse with each repetition.

step by step

1. Lie on your back with your knees bent into your chest and open shoulder-width apart and your heels squeezed tightly together.
2. Layer hands behind the base of your head and pull your powerhouse down toward the mat to secure your lower back.
3. Lift your head and look toward your powerhouse.
4. Inhale, deepening the scoop in your powerhouse, and press your legs away from you.
5. Exhale and bring your knees back toward your shoulders, creating imagined resistance.
6. *Imagine you are pulling in a heavy spring that's attached to the wall in front of you.*
7. Repeat 5 to 8 times. End by lowering your head to the mat and stretching your body out to full length to prepare for the Roll Up.

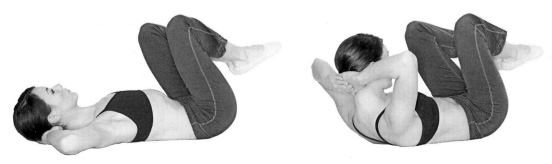

strengthens abs and inner
thighs, stretches shoulders

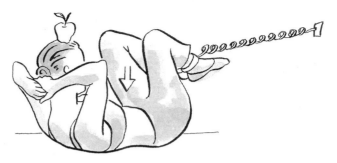

do

- Keep your upper body perfectly still, *as if balancing an apple on your head*.
- Continue to squeeze your heels together to work your inner thighs and maintain alignment.
- Press your shoulder blades deeply into the mat beneath you to secure your position.
- Keep your elbows as wide as possible throughout the movement.

don't

- Do not bend your leg without pulling from the powerhouse.
- Do not allow your bottom to lift off the mat.

modification: Place hands in a V shape under your bottom to support the lower back.

progression: Before pulling your knees back in, keep your extended legs long and point and flex your feet while holding your inhalation.

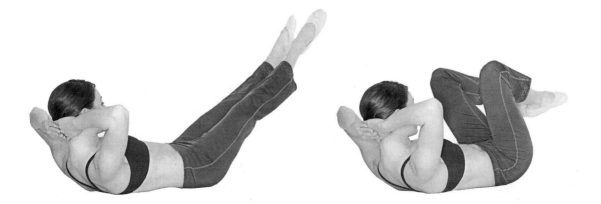

STOMACH MASSAGE I

goal: To keep lifting out of your lower back throughout movement while deepening your powerhouse.

step by step

Transition from the Roll Up by rolling up to sitting and drawing your knees into your chest with your heels together and tiptoes touching the mat.

1. Lift your feet off the floor and balance on your tailbone with your knees bent into your chest shoulder-width apart, and with your arms encircling your thighs.
2. Stay lifted and look to your powerhouse without dropping your head forward.
3. *Imagine you are balanced on a thumbtack.*
4. Inhale and stretch your legs up into the air without changing your upper body form. Your heels stay glued together throughout.
5. Exhale as you flex your feet hard; inhale as you point them.
6. Pull your knees back into your chest, pressing all the air from your lungs as you do. *Imagine squeezing the air from a balloon between your thighs and chest.*
7. Repeat 5 to 8 times. End by rolling down to the mat with your knees bent into your chest and arms at right angles by your sides to prepare for the Coordination.

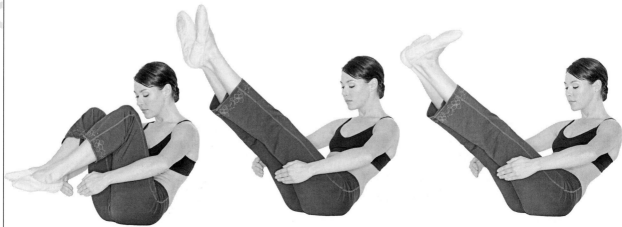

firms abs and arms, stretches and
strengthens feet

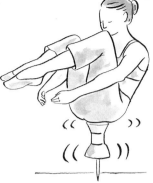

do

- Keep your legs "light" by focusing your movements on drawing your belly in and up.
- Keep your heels squeezed tightly together throughout movement.
- Stay long in the neck. *Imagine balancing books on your head* as you perform the sequence.

don't

- Don't roll forward. Stay balanced on your tailbone.
- Don't allow your knees to fall open. *Imagine holding a ball between your knees.*
- Don't drop your feet. Instead try to "pull" your knees toward your shoulders with control.

modification: Do not hold the extended position to point and flex feet. Simply stretch and bend your legs with control and concentration. Place your fingertips on the mat for balance.

progression: Hold your arms overhead throughout, with your elbows open to the sides and your shoulders rolling down and back.

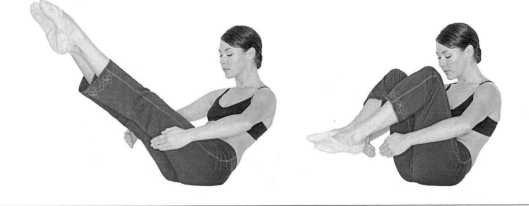

COORDINATION

goal: Fluid movement with attention to full exhalations.

step by step

1. Lie on your back with your knees bent into your chest and open hip-width apart and your heels squeezed together tightly.
2. Lift your head and look to your powerhouse. Bend your elbows and hold them tightly to your sides at a 90-degree angle.
3. Inhale, deepening the scoop in your powerhouse, and press your legs and arms away from you.
4. Hold your breath as you open and close your legs.
5. Exhale fully as you bring your knees back toward your shoulders, creating imagined resistance.
6. *Imagine deflating a ball with your knees as you pull them in. Squeeze all the air from the ball.*
7. When you're at the end of your exhalation, bend your elbows and return to the starting position. Keep your heels lifted throughout.
8. Repeat 5 to 8 times. End by rolling up to sitting for Rolling Like a Ball.

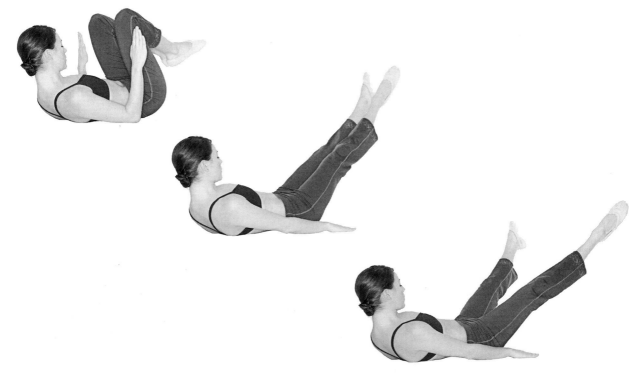

increases ab strength, lung capacity
and tones inner thighs

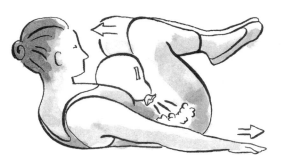

do

- Open and close your legs from the outer and inner thigh rather than working from the feet. *Imagine a band wrapped around your outer thighs that you must press apart and resist to close your legs.*
- Use the inward pull of your knees to cleanse your lungs of stale air.
- Reach your arms farther forward as you pull your knees in, creating opposition and working the sides of the body.

don't

- Do not allow your lower back to arch up off the mat as you press your legs away.
- Do not allow your shoulders to curl up around your ears. Pin your elbows to the mat.

modification: Place your hands in a V shape under your bottom to support your lower back and perform with the legs only until you are able to add the arm movements.

progression: With your legs extended, perform a small ballet *changement* crossing the right leg slightly over left, then the left over the right, switching 8 times while sustaining the inhalation; then pull your knees back into your chest and exhale.

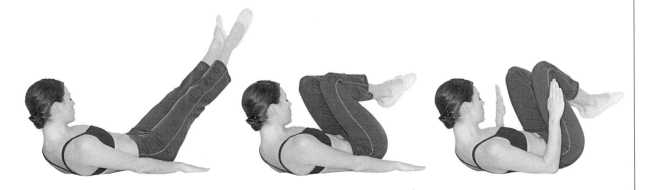

R O W I N G   I

goal: To stay long in your lower back throughout the entire sequence.

step by step

Transition from Rolling Like a Ball by releasing your ankles and straightening your legs out on the mat in front of you.

1. Sit tall with your legs extended in the Pilates stance, and pull your fists into your breast bone. Stretch your elbows wide to the sides.
2. Inhale as you roll backward, scooping your belly toward the mat and squeezing the backs of your inner thighs together for stability.
3. Draw your fists back with you, and stop where you can manage to hold yourself steady. Stretch your legs in opposition with your heels firmly planted on the mat.
4. Holding still with your powerhouse, open your arms out wide to your sides with your palms facing back.
5. Exhale and bring your upper body through your arms. *Imagine your arms are heavy oars with which you are rowing.* Allow your hands to come together at your tailbone as you stretch forward.
6. Inhale and slowly lift your hands upward, stretching your arms toward the ceiling. Do *not* allow your shoulders to "pop" as you perform this stretch!
7. Exhale as you circle your arms around to your feet in a sweeping motion.
8. *Imagine lifting your body forward as a champion butterflyer would to win a swimming race.*
9. Roll up to your starting position and repeat the sequence 3 to 5 times. End by pulling one knee into your chest and slowly rolling down to the mat for the Single Leg Stretch.

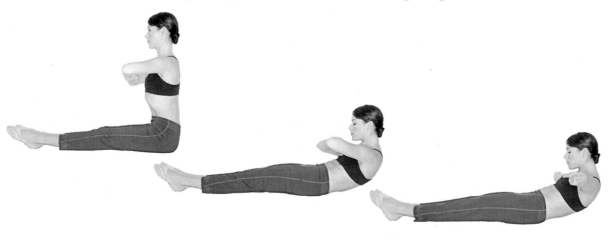

strengthens abs, stretches shoulders
and lower back

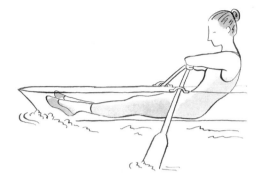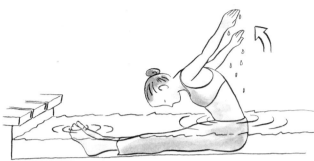

do

- Keep your buttocks and legs engaged throughout.
- Create resistance in your powerhouse as you stretch forward to enhance the stretch.
- Lengthen the front of your thighs in opposition to your powerhouse as you roll back.

don't

- Do not allow your shoulders to ride up around your ears at any stage in the exercise.
- Do not allow your shoulders to overrotate or pop.

modification: Bend both knees and place your feet flat on the mat two feet from your bottom. Use your hands on the underside of your thighs for support and roll back to the mat on an inhalation; then exhale as you roll up and over, knees straightening in the process. Bring your hands to your tailbone and complete steps 6 to 8. Finish by rolling up to sitting with bent knees (repeat the sequence 3 to 5 times).

progression: Try to roll your entire back down onto the mat as if lying down, without disengaging your powerhouse.

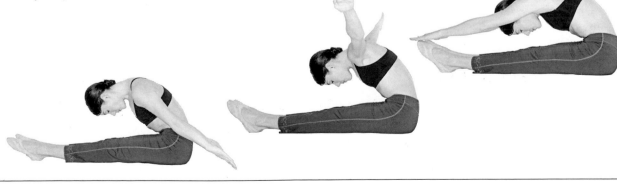

LONG STRETCH

goal: To keep powerhouse engaged and pulled up into your spine. Fight gravity!

step by step

Transition from the Open Leg Rocker by closing your legs and bending your knees. Twist your upper body to the side, and put your palms on the mat—let your lower body follow until you have pressed up onto hands and knees. (*Advanced transition:* Close your legs in the rocker position and, with straight legs, twist toward mat and transition directly into a push-up position.)

1. Begin on your hands and knees.
2. Make sure your hands are directly underneath your shoulders and curl your toes under. Pull your navel up into your spine as you stretch one leg out at a time until you are in a push-up position.
3. Squeeze the backs of your legs and make sure your body is held in a straight line—don't let the hips sink.
4. *Imagine you are as strong and straight as a battering ram.*
5. Inhale as you rock forward onto the balls of your feet.
6. Exhale as you shift your body weight backward, pressing your heels toward the mat.
7. Repeat 5 times and then bend knees and lower your body down to mat to prepare for the Double Leg Kick. (*Advanced transition:* Lower your whole body to the mat from a push-up position.)

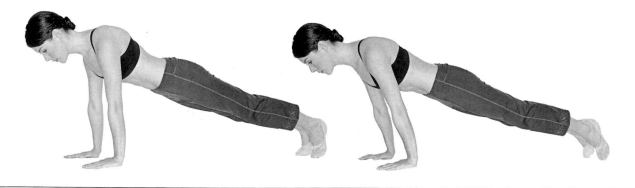

strengthens abs, arms, legs, and buttocks

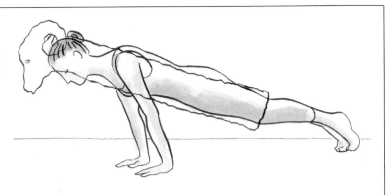

do

- Keep legs squeezing together tightly to stabilize your lower body.
- Push the floor away from you with your arms to maintain lift in the body.
- Lengthen the back of your neck and lead with the crown of your head.

don't

- Do not lock elbows. Keep a very slight outward rotation in your elbows to ensure that your arm muscles are working, you are not just resting on your joints, and that the movements are coming from the sides of the body.
- Do not sink into your back or shoulders.

modification: Perform the exercise propped up on your elbows. Make sure you begin with your elbows slightly forward of your shoulders and keep your hands (or fists) pressing into the mat. Do not sink into your shoulders at any stage.

progression: Lift one leg slightly off the mat and hold it in the air as you rock back and forward 3 times. Switch legs. Use the same breathing pattern as described at left.

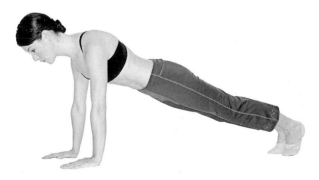

REFORMER TEASER

goal: To use the arm circles as tools to lengthen out of your lower back and waist.

step by step

Transition from the Low Back Stretch by rolling up to sitting and turning your upper body to place your palms on the mat to one side. Press through your palms and lift your bottom up, twisting it underneath you until you are sitting. Roll your back down to the mat.

1. Lie on your back with your knees bent into your chest, and your arms stretched long by your sides, palms up. Squeeze your heels together tightly and open knees hip-width apart.
2. Lift your head up and forward to look toward your powerhouse.
3. Inhale and begin rolling up to sitting, as you simultaneously straighten your legs to a 45-degree angle and hold them in Pilates stance.
4. Exhale and hold, squeezing your legs together tightly, until no light comes through them.
5. Continue to balance on your tail as you slowly draw 3 forward circles with your arms, trying to lift higher out of your lower back with each circle. Inhale to begin each circle and exhale to complete it.
6. *Imagine circling your arms with resistance, as if you were holding heavy paint cans.* Circle with concentration and control, *so as to not spill a drop.*
7. Hold your arms up on the final circle, sustaining the inhalation, and then slowly exhale as you roll your spine down to the mat with control, bringing your body back to the starting position.
8. Repeat 3 to 5 times.

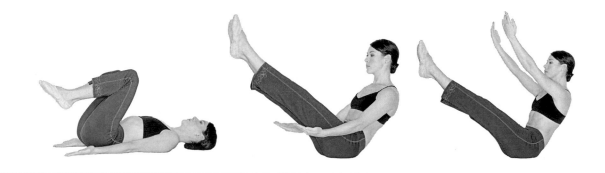

tightens waistline and inner thighs,
tones arms and shoulders

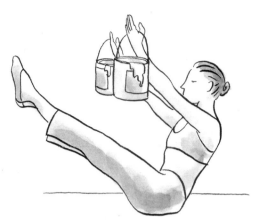

do

- Initiate each circle with a lift in the powerhouse and allow your arms to follow that lift.
- Keep your palms up and reaching for the ceiling.
- Keep your gaze lifted and shoulders pressing down away from your ears.

don't

- Do not lock your elbows. Keep a very slight outward rotation in your elbows to ensure that the movements are coming from the sides of the body. *Imagine having a heavy pile of laundry in your arms.*
- Do not allow your shoulders to lift at any stage of the exercise.
- Do not lean back so far as to sink into your lower back.

modification: Keep your knees slightly bent throughout the exercise sequence.

progression: Keep your arms lifted above your head as you roll up into the position and back down. Do not allow your shoulders to engage.

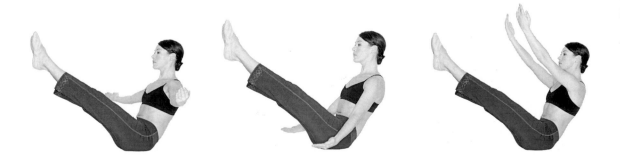

Lean Lower Body

Contrary to common belief, toning your lower body (as I define it: hips, thighs, and buttocks) and getting the long, lean look you want cannot be achieved by pounding the pavement or loading up on iron plates at the gym, but rather by stretching and activating muscle groups to create length. The Lean Lower Body series uses movements that force you to work in longer, more outstretched positions and to increase joint flexibility and range of motion. The more you can imagine incorporating oppositional stretch into these exercises, the better the results will be.

note: The Tantalizing Ten exercises are shown in the road map to indicate their placement within the new series. The instructions in the following pages pertain to the new Lean Lower Body exercises. I have slotted the new movements into the places I deem appropriate to keep the proper rhythm and flow of the matwork. In Pilates you are never in one position for too long and in keeping with that philosophy and its related cardio results, I have sewn each new exercise into the fabric of the Tantalizing Ten as seamlessly as possible. Instructions on each page will transition you to and from exercise to exercise. Remember to stay focused on your goal of lengthening your lower body throughout the execution of each movement without forsaking your powerhouse. This will make all the difference in the effects Pilates has on your body.

road map

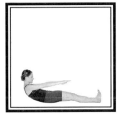

roll up
beginner

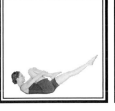

long strap circles
advanced

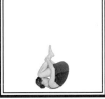

rolling like a ball
beginner

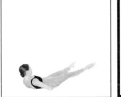

single leg stretch
beginner

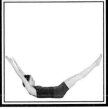

double leg stretch
intermediate

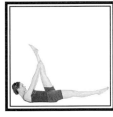

single straight leg
stretch
intermediate

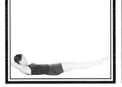

double straight leg
stretch
advanced

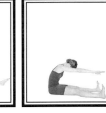

crisscross
advanced

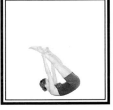

spine stretch
forward
beginner

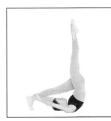

open leg rocker
intermediate

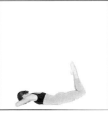

balance/control
very advanced

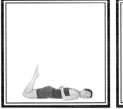

grasshopper
advanced

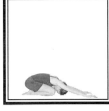

double leg kick
advanced

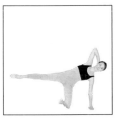

low back stretch

kneeling side circles
advanced

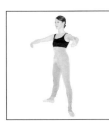

gondola
intermediate

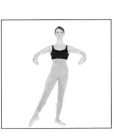

standing leg press
intermediate

LONG STRAP CIRCLES

goal: To deepen the powerhouse with each repetition.

step by step

Transition from the Roll Up by remaining on your back and bringing your arms down to your sides.

1. Lie on your back with your hands under your bottom (see detail page 85) and legs at 90 degrees in the Pilates stance. Lift your head and look to your powerhouse.
2. Inhale, deepening the scoop in your powerhouse, and begin to circle your legs open and down. Stop when you can no longer maintain a flat back. *Imagine your upper body is strapped to the mat.*
3. Exhale and bring your legs together and back up to your starting position.
4. Repeat 5 to 8 times and then hug knees into your chest. Place your feet flat on the floor, squeeze your legs together, and roll up to sitting for Rolling Like a Ball.

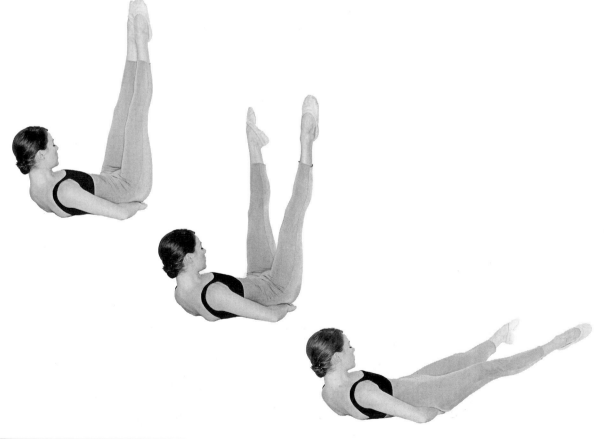

strengthens abs, slims hips
and inner thighs

do

- Keep your upper body perfectly still, *as if a great weight were sitting on your chest.*
- Press your shoulder blades deep into the mat to secure your position.
- Keep your elbows as wide as possible throughout the movement to help keep your shoulders down.

don't

- Do not open your legs so wide that you cannot control the movement.
- Do not allow your bottom to lift off the mat as you bring your legs up to 90 degrees.
- Do not allow your shoulder blades to lift off the mat as you lower your legs.
- Do not arch in your lower back.

modification: Keep your head down and make small circles with your legs at 90 degrees.

progression: Layer your hands behind the base of your head and still maintain a flat back as you perform the exercise.

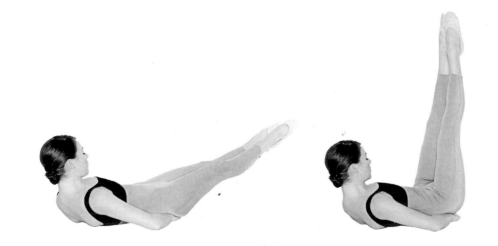

BALANCE/CONTROL

goal: To maintain a stable upper body while rhythmically working the length of your legs.

note: *Very* advanced. Make sure you can do the Modification safely before doing the full exercise.

step by step

Transition from the Open Leg Rocker by closing your legs and rolling your back down to the mat without moving your legs. Bring your arms overhead.

1. Lie on your back with your arms overhead and legs at 90 degrees in the Pilates stance.
2. Inhale as you roll your legs overhead, initiating the lift from your powerhouse, and bring your feet to your hands.
3. Make sure that you are balanced on the back of your shoulders and *not* on your neck!
4. Hold left ankle with both hands, curling the toes of your left foot under, and extend the right leg straight up to the ceiling as high as possible, *as if unfolding a jointed ruler.*
5. Release your ankle and switch legs without changing any part of your form.
6. *Imagine pulling a rubber band apart between your ankles throughout.*
7. Complete 3 to 5 sets and then bring both legs up into the air and slowly roll down your spine, away from your fingertips, articulating your spine for a deep spinal stretch.
8. Lower your legs to the mat (bend them if you need to) and roll onto your stomach, resting your forehead on the backs of your hands to prepare for the Grasshopper.

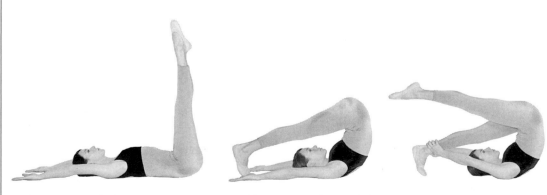

stretches back muscles
and firms bottom

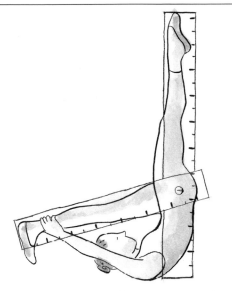

do

- Initiate your switch with the bottom leg. Do not drop your top leg to execute the movement.
- Engage your buttocks with each lift and open the front of your hip by trying to touch the ceiling with your extending foot.

don't

- Do *not* roll all your weight onto your neck at any point in the exercise!
- Do not drop your raised leg even 1 inch until your other leg meets it.

modification: Perform only one slow set, without lifting your arms overhead. Instead, press your arms long on the mat along your sides. Do *not* roll weight onto your neck!

progression: Press your arms down on the mat along your sides and make the rhythm as dynamic as in the Single Straight Leg Stretch (p. 96). Do *not* roll onto your neck!

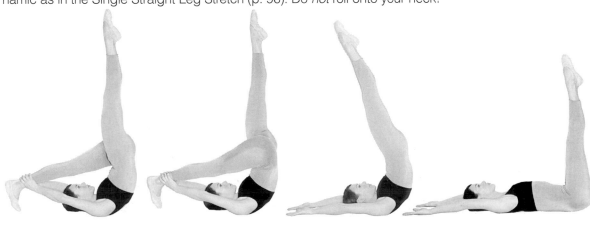

GRASSHOPPER

goal: To keep your knees lifted as high off of mat as possible throughout the lifted portion without straining your lower back.

step by step

1. Lie on your stomach with your forehead resting on your layered hands and your legs squeezing together in the Pilates stance.
2. Inhale, pulling your tummy up into your spine, and raise your legs up off of the mat (including your thighs!) *as if your legs were suspended from the ceiling.*
3. Hold your breath as you bring your heels to your bottom; then straighten them back out again, keeping your knees up off the mat throughout (you may allow your knees to open into a diamond shape, but your heels stay glued together for alignment).
4. *Imagine you are squeezing a ball between your heels and bottom;* use resistance.
5. Exhale as you lower your straight legs beating them together quickly (*as if clapping*) as you go.
6. Repeat 5 times and then bring your hands behind your back and turn your face to one side resting your cheek on the mat to prepare for Double Leg Kicks.

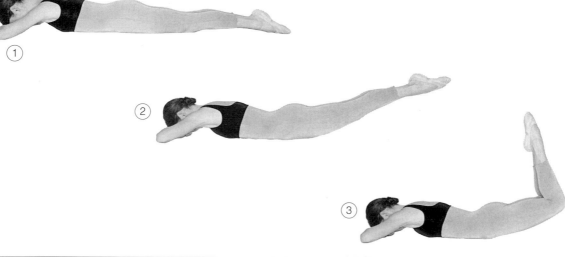

LEAN LOWER BODY ADVANCED

strengthens lower back and buttocks,
stretches hips, thighs, and abs

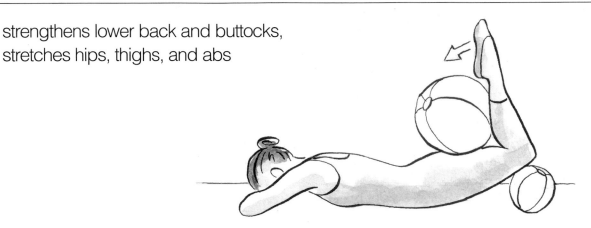

do

- When beating, use your entire leg, not just the heels, and feel the work in the inner thighs.

don't

- Do not throw your legs into the air, lift them with control.

modification: Perform only the lifting and lowering of the legs without kicking your bottom. Add the clapping portion when your back feels strong.

progression: Keep your legs squeezing together in parallel throughout (all but the clapping portion of the exercise).

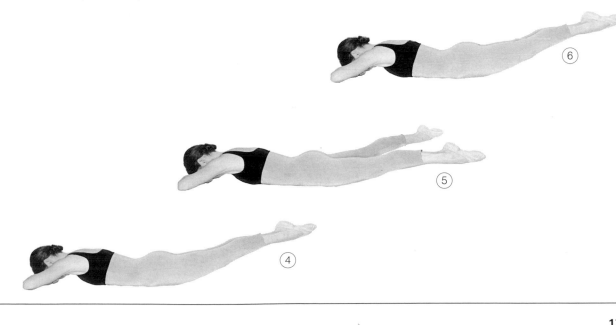

KNEELING SIDE CIRCLES

goal: To anchor your body's frame while keeping your circling leg "light."

step by step

Transition from the Low Back Stretch by rolling up to a kneeling position.

1. Kneel on your mat and prop yourself up on one hand to your side, making sure it is aligned directly beneath your shoulder. Place the heel of your opposite hand on the side of your head and press the side of your head gently into it to maintain proper neck and spine alignment.
2. Reach your top leg out long on the mat and then lift it to hip height, turning it out slightly to engage your buttocks.
3. Stabilize your shoulders and hips, *as if they were two Corinthian columns.*
4. Inhale and begin drawing a forward circle with your leg on the opposite wall, exhale to complete the circle.
5. *Imagine carving circles into wet plaster on the wall.*
6. Complete 3 to 5 circles in one direction and then switch directions for 3 to 5 circles.
7. Bring your knee back to the starting position and lift your body upright.
8. Repeat the sequence to the other side. End in an upright kneeling position. Place one foot flat on the mat in front of you and then step directly up into the Pilates stance in preparation for the Gondola. (*Advanced transition:* Curl your toes underneath you, lean back, and lift up to standing from a kneeling position without separating your legs. Use your arms for leverage.)

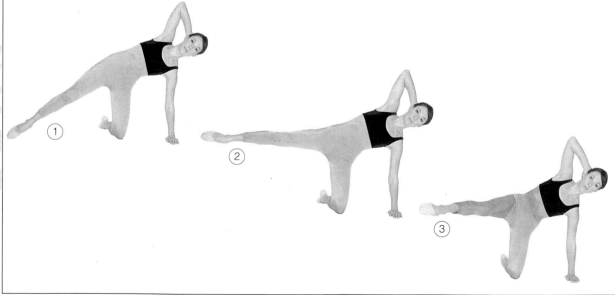

tightens waistline and buttocks,
strengthens upper back

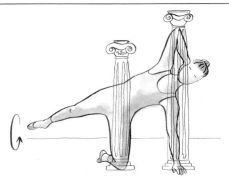

do

- Keep cinching up in your waistline to help take pressure off the supporting wrist.
- Keep a slight turnout in your circling leg to work your buttocks and the back of your thigh.
- Stay square in your body, making sure to keep your hip directly over the bent knee.
- Continually deepen the scoop in your powerhouse while pushing your pubic bone forward.
- Keep the crown of your head reaching in opposition to your circling leg.

don't

- Do not grip with your thigh muscle to circle. Use your buttocks and the back of your leg.
- Do not allow your head to drop. Press it up into your hand to help strengthen your neck.
- Avoid locking your knee to lengthen the leg. Stretch your leg from your hip and waistline.
- Do not "break" at your hip and allow your buttocks to move backward. Continually push your bottom forward to stretch the front of your hip and thigh.

modification: Lift and lower your leg without circling.

progression: Increase the diameter of the circles without losing balance or changing form.

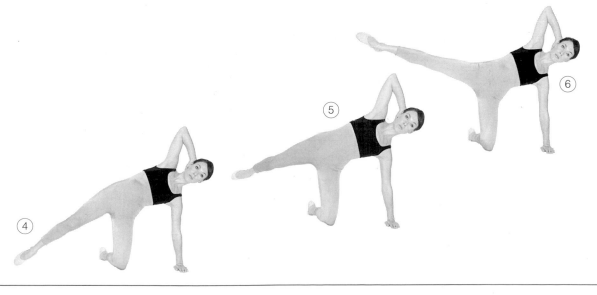

G O N D O L A

goal: To stay light on your feet by lifting your waistline.

step by step

1. Stand with your legs and feet turned out wider than the Pilates stance, but not so much as to cause strain in your knees. Make sure that the turn out is originating from your hips and *not* from your feet. Squeeze your inner thighs and buttocks tightly together and press your pubic bone forward. Pull up deeply in your powerhouse to fight gravity.
2. Hold your arms open with elbows lifted to engage and tone the backs of your arms.
3. Inhale and slide your right foot out to the side with balance and control, *as if on roller skates.*
4. Hold your inhalation as you bend deeply at the knees, making sure that your knees are open over your baby toes.
5. Exhale as you slide your right heel to meet your left, still maintain the bend in your knees.
6. Continue to exhale as you push into your heels to stand up, *as if zipping up your legs.*
7. Complete 3 to 5 repetitions and then reverse the movements:
8. Standing in the Pilates stance, inhale as you bend your knees deeply, making sure your knees are directly over your baby toes.
9. Hold your inhalation as you slide your left foot away from your right and shift your weight so that it is evenly balanced. Maintain your knee bend throughout.
10. Exhale as you straighten your legs without locking them.
11. Continue the exhalation as you shift your weight, as slightly as possible, to the right in order to slide your left leg to meet your right leg. Initiate this slide from the lift in your powerhouse.
12. Complete 3 to 5 repetitions. End in the Pilates stance to prepare for the Standing Leg Press.

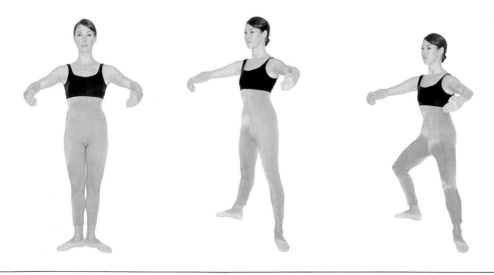

134

tones arms, stretches hips, and
flattens abs

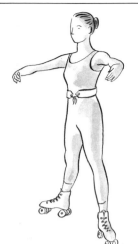

do

- Initiate each movement from your powerhouse muscles and leave your legs light.
- Keep your open knees as pressed back as possible.
- Keep a long lower back (you may feel like you need to curl your pelvis up under you a bit).

don't

- Do not lock your knees at any point in the exercise or let them roll inward.
- Do not allow your bottom to stick out behind you.

modification: Simply perform 5 to 8 deep knee bends with your heels together and then 5 to 8 knee bends with your heels apart to work on your standing form and the opening of your hips.

progression: Perform the entire sequence on the balls of your feet. Do *not* put pressure out over your toes. If possible, hold on to a wall in front of you for stability as you practice. (Note: Make this easier by wearing socks.)

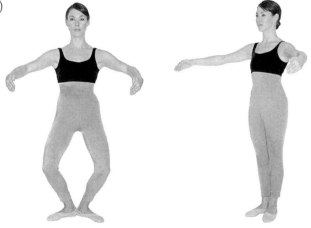

STANDING LEG PRESS

goal: To use each leg press to lift and lengthen your waistline.

step by step

1. Stand in Pilates stance with your arms open and elbows lifted to engage and tone the backs of your arms.
2. Pulling up deeply in your powerhouse lift your right foot 1 to 2 feet off the ground. Your big toe is on line with your belly button and your inner thigh faces the ceiling.
3. Growing taller, inhale and press your leg and foot down with imagined resistance, *as if pulling on a spring attached to the wall in front of you.*
4. Hold for a count of 3, then use your exhalation to lift the leg up with lightness and control.
5. Do 3 to 5 presses and then switch legs. Repeat steps 1 to 4 with your left leg.
6. After the last repetition to the front, switch legs again, this time bringing your right leg out to the side and holding it 1 to 2 feet off the ground and slightly forward of your right hip.
7. Growing taller, inhale and press your leg and foot down with imagined resistance, *as if pulling on a spring attached to the wall to the side of you.*
8. Hold for a count of 3, then use your exhalation to lift the leg up with lightness and control.
9. Repeat 3 to 5 presses and then return to standing to switch legs. Repeat steps 6 to 8 with left leg.
10. After the last repetition to the side, switch your legs again, this time bringing your right leg out behind you and holding it 1 to 2 feet off the ground and in line with your right hip.
11. Growing taller, inhale and press your leg and foot down with imagined resistance, *as if pulling on a spring attached to the wall behind you.*
12. Hold for a count of 3, then use your exhalation to lift the leg up with lightness and control.
13. Repeat 3 to 5 presses and then switch legs. Repeat steps 10 to 12 with your left leg.

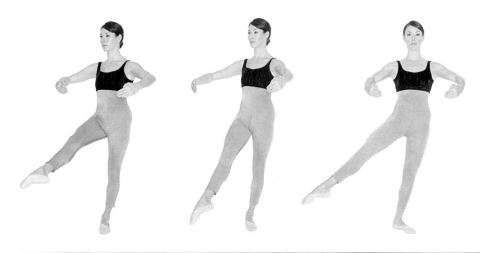

136

firms arms and buttocks,
improves balance

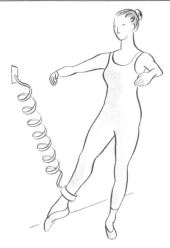

do

- Make sure you create enough resistance with your mind to elicit the results you desire.
- Perform the entire sequence, front, side, and back, without dropping into your waist or hips.
- Make sure your body is square and your standing leg is directly beneath your hip.

don't

- Do not allow your shoulders to lift as you maintain lifted elbows.
- Do not lift leg too high. Focus on the press—not the height—and lengthening the waist.
- Do not lock your standing knee joint or place weight in your standing heel.
- Do not allow your lower back to arch when lifting your leg behind you.

modification: Try simply lifting each extended leg and then placing it down on the floor, using the floor as a pedal to push down on. Repeat this 3 times, growing taller with each press.

progression: At steps 4, 8, and 12 leave leg lifted and pulse it 3 times, *as if bouncing a ball in the air.*

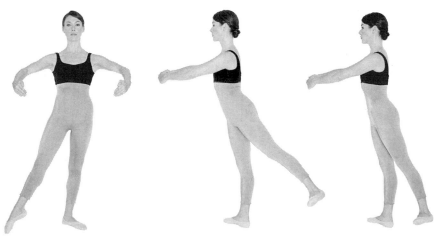

Perfecting Posture

Good posture is made up of a series of combined elements: strong spinal muscles, flexibility in the chest and shoulders, and strong abdominals and neck along with muscular balance and a good range of motion in your joints. In many ways posture begins at, and can be traced right down to, your toes. Poor posture causes muscular strain and therefore wastes energy. It can also cause crowding of the internal organs resulting in impaired function. It produces imbalanced stress on spinal joints and discs and, in extreme cases, can even cause permanent damage. In the Perfecting Posture series you will be using exercises specifically designed to stretch and strengthen the target muscle groups and create the balance so essential to maintaining a poised and graceful you. Remember to take these postural lessons with you off the mat and adapt them into your gym, sports, and Invisible Workout® routines. Most of all, stay continually aware of your posture throughout the day. This awareness can be the very catalyst to improving your posture without delay.

note: The Tantalizing Ten exercises are shown on the road map to indicate their placement within the new series. The instructions in the following pages pertain to the new Perfecting Posture exercises. I have slotted the new movements into the places I deem appropriate to keep the proper rhythm and flow of the matwork. In Pilates you are never in one position for too long and in keeping with that philosophy and its related cardio results, I have sewn each new exercise into the fabric of the Tantalizing Ten as seamlessly as possible. Instructions on each page will transition you from exercise to exercise. Remember to stay focused on your goal of perfecting your posture as you execute each movement. Recalibrate the exercises of the Tantalizing Ten to suit your goal of perfect posture as well. If you think it, it will come!

road map

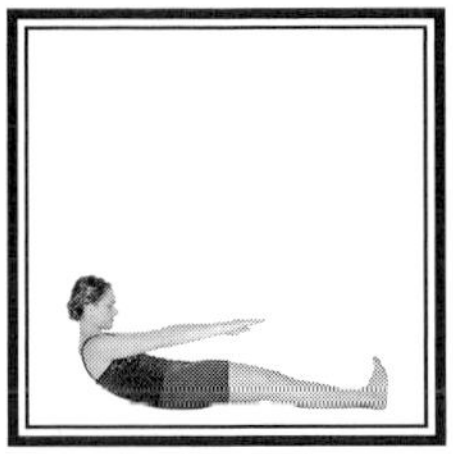

roll up
beginner

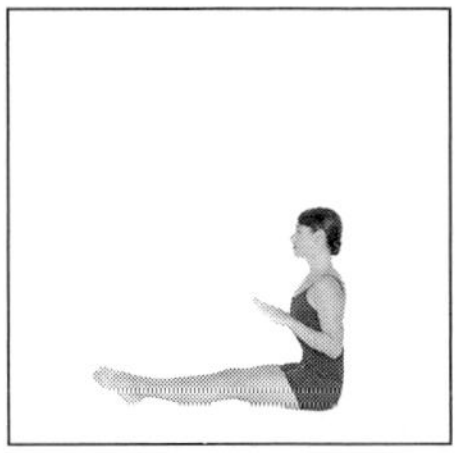

rowing from chest
intermediate

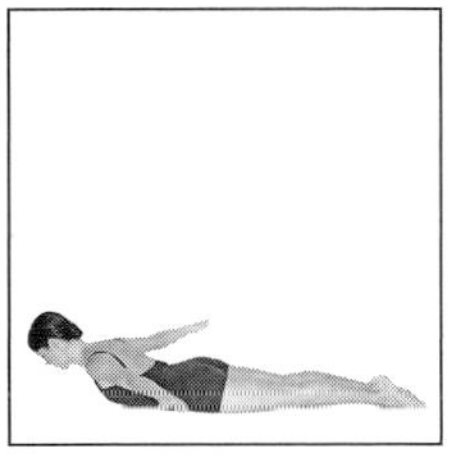

pull straps II
advanced

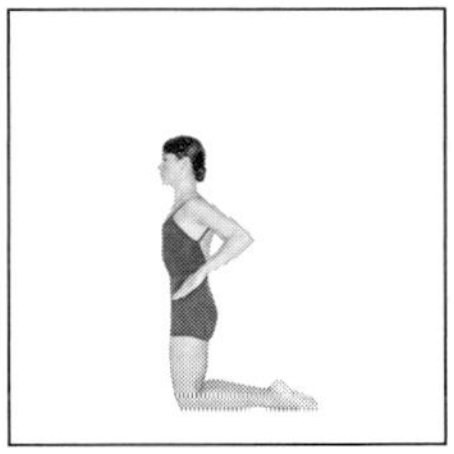

long back stretch
intermediate

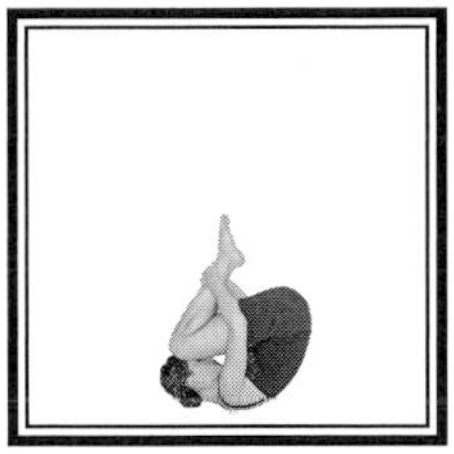

rolling like a ball
beginner

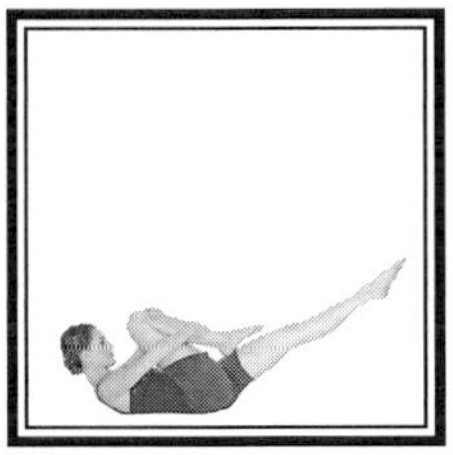

single leg stretch
beginner

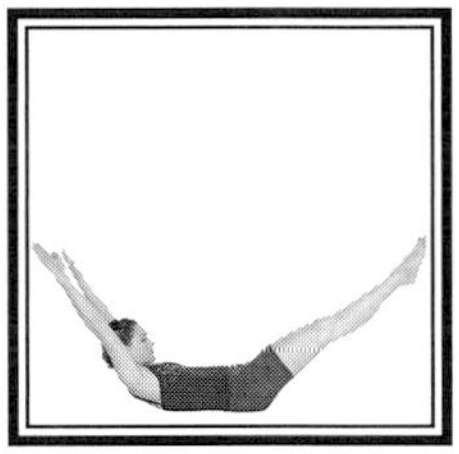

double leg stretch
intermediate

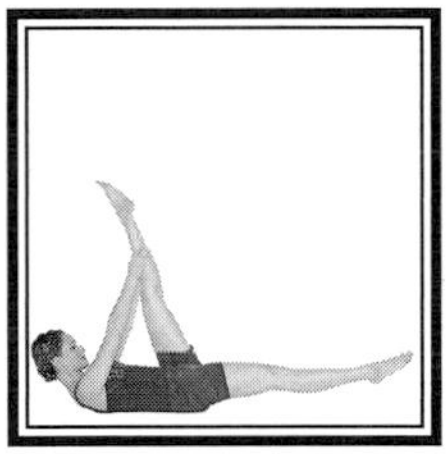

single straight leg
stretch
intermediate

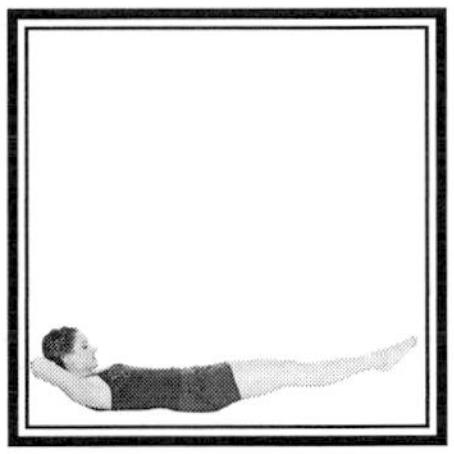

double straight leg
stretch
advanced

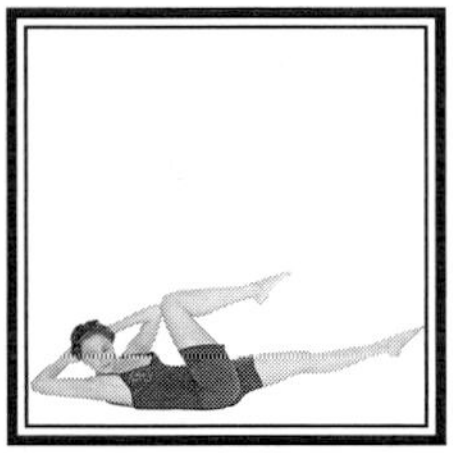

crisscross
advanced

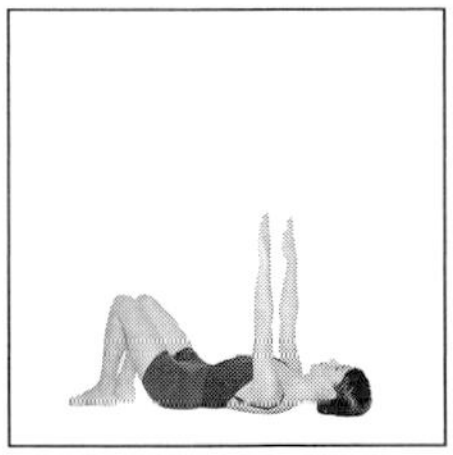

the breathing
beginner

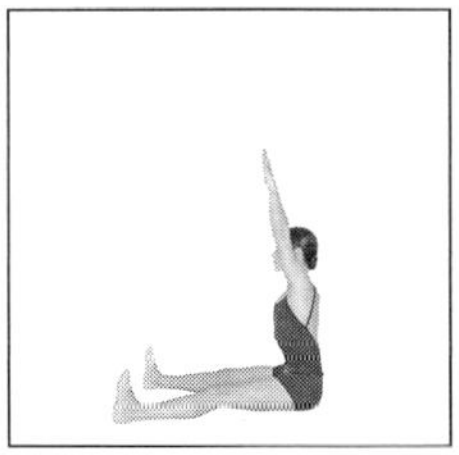

spine stretch with
arm circles
beginner

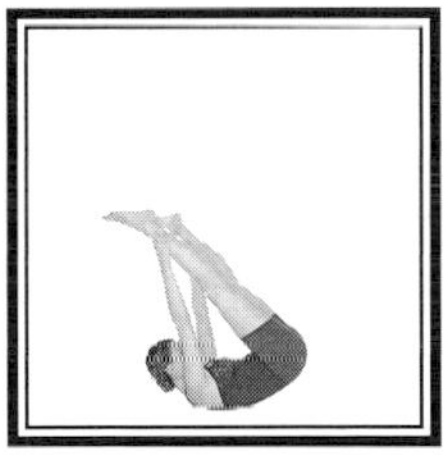

open leg rocker
intermediate

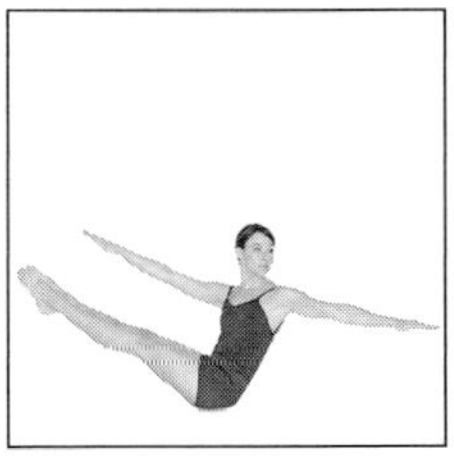

stomach
massage III
advanced

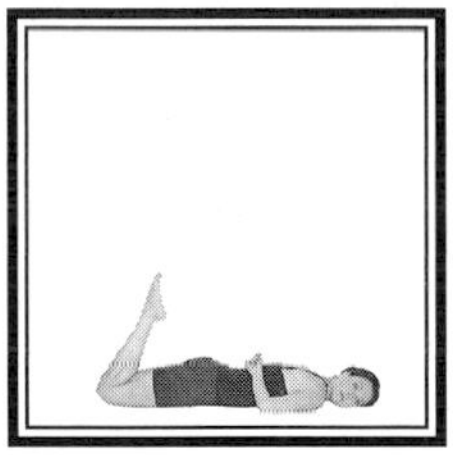

double leg kick
advanced

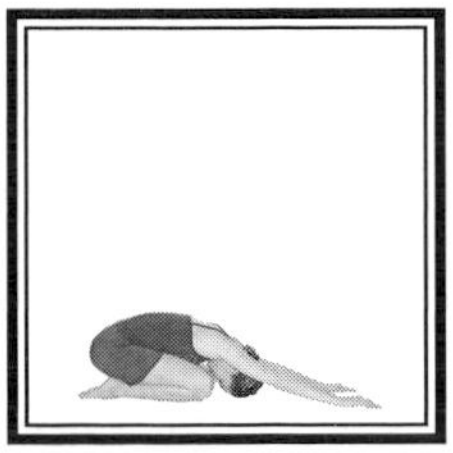

low back stretch

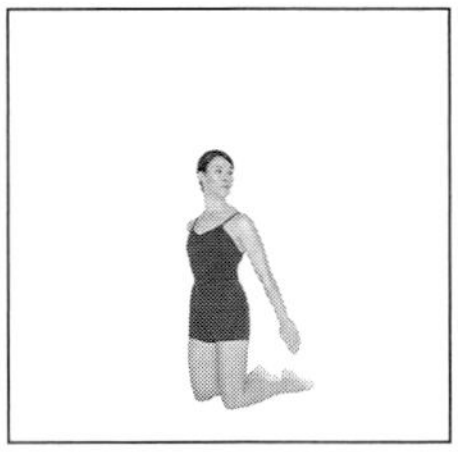

chest expansion
intermediate

ROWING FROM CHEST

goal: To use the movement of your arms to lift you up in your waist.

step by step

Transition from the Roll Up by rolling up to sitting with your arms by your sides.

1. Sit tall with your legs extended and in the Pilates stance in front of you, feet long and relaxed, and your elbows bent tightly into your sides with palms down and fingers extended.
2. Inhale as you sit taller and stretch your arms out, bringing your body into a slight forward pitch to stretch your lower back, *as if you were being pulled up and away by a jumbo jet.*
3. Keep your shoulders low, exhale, and press your arms down until fingertips touch the mat.
4. Inhale as you lift your arms up to the ceiling in one swift movement, feeling your waistline lift with your rising arms—but keeping your ribs pulled in. Keep your shoulders pressing down, creating opposition.
5. Grow taller and as you slowly exhale, press your arms out to the sides with strong resistance, *as if you were a gymnast performing on the rings.*
6. As your hands near the mat bend your arms and pull them back tightly into your sides.
7. Complete 3 to 5 repetitions and turn over onto your belly. Lie face down with your arms out-stretched to the sides in preparation for the Pull Straps II.

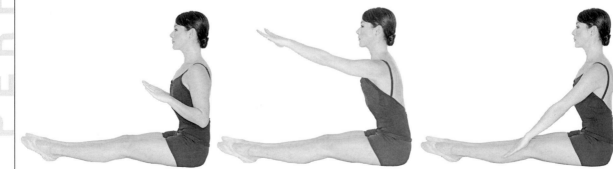

tightens waistline, defines shoulders,
increases lung capacity

do

- Reach your arms toward either side on the room as you press down to engage your "wings."
- Engage your inner thighs throughout by squeezing them together, to create stability.

don't

- Do not allow your arms to move behind your shoulders when you circle them down. Keep them within your periphery.
- Do not lock your elbows or grip with your knees.

modification: Bend your knees and place your feet flat on the mat, hip-width apart with your heels 2 feet from your bottom. Perform the rowing sequence as described.

progression: As you bring your arms around place your palms flat on the mat and bow your head to your knees. Exhale as you slide your hands along the mat to your heels with your head still on your knees. Inhale as you roll up to sitting with your arms outstretched in front of you at shoulder height. Exhale as you bend your elbows back into your sides and repeat the entire rowing sequence.

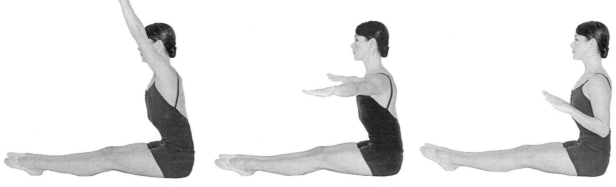

PULL STRAPS II

goal: To secure your lower body so your upper body can move freely.

step by step

1. Lie on your stomach with your arms stretched out to your sides, your forehead on the mat and neck long. Make sure that your tummy is pulled up into your spine and that your legs are squeezing together in the Pilates stance with buttocks tight.
2. Inhale as you lift your chest and arms up off the mat and reach your arms behind you in one controlled step. Move your arms back through the air with resistance, opening the fronts of your shoulders and engaging the backs of your arms, *as if you were opening giant wings.*
3. Sustain your inhalation, keeping your chest lifted.
4. *Imagine you are being pulled backward by a giant parachute.*
5. At the count of 3 slowly begin exhaling as your reverse the movements, lowering yourself down to the mat. Lead from your chest and then follow with your arms.
6. Complete 5 repetitions and then sit back to your heels in the Low Back Stretch. Roll up to sit on your heels and then lift your bottom up and into a kneeling position to prepare for the Long Back Stretch.

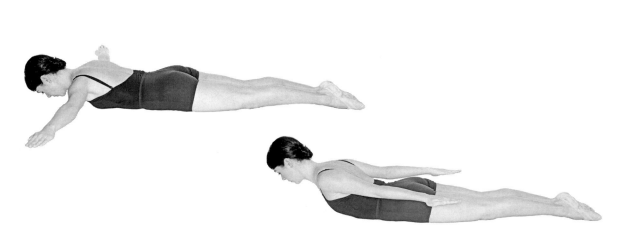

strengthens arms and upper back,
firms buttocks, increases lung
capacity

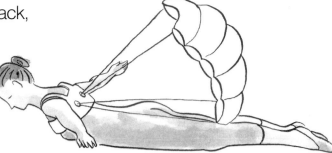

do

- Press shoulders away from crown of your head to create length in the back of your neck.
- Stretch the crown of your head away from your heels to lengthen and protect your lower back.
- Engage the muscles in the backs of your upper arms by reaching them for each other and stretching your fingertips toward your heels as they reach back.
- Engage the muscles in your upper back and shoulders by reaching your arms for opposing walls as you bring them back to your starting position.

don't

- Do not throw your arms backward to initiate the lift in your chest.
- Do not arch your lower back but secure the muscles by tightening your abdominals.
- Do not allow your head to fall backward or crunch into the back of your neck.
- Do not allow your heels to come apart throughout the exercise.

modification: Perform the arm movements without lifting your head and chest off of the mat. Be sure to initiate the arm sequence by engaging your powerhouse and securing your leg position.

progression: Start with your arms reaching forward (as in Pilates Swimming, p. 204), and perform the sequence but return to the new position each time. Do not allow your shoulders to climb up to your ears.

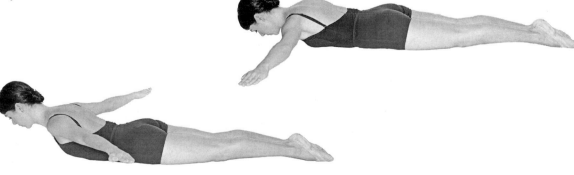

LONG BACK STRETCH

goal: To use the movement of your arms to increase the lift in your chest.

step by step

1. Kneel on your mat with your legs squeezing together, buttocks tight and arms reaching long by your sides. Keep your pubic bone pressing forward to open the fronts of your hips.
2. Inhaling, pull your powerhouse in deeply and press both arms back—with resistance—as far as you are able, lifting your chest in opposition to your elbows.
3. Maintaining your inhalation, bend your arms lifting your elbows as high as possible behind you as you bring your hands up to chest height, palms face down and fingers extended. Your arms are squeezing in tightly to your sides.
4. *Imagine your upper arms being pulled up and back.*
5. Press your palms straight down toward the mat with resistance, *as if hoisting yourself up on two invisible chairs.* Press the crown of your head to the ceiling in opposition to your fingertips.
6. Complete 3 to 5 repetitions and then reverse the sequence for 3 to 5 additional stretches. End by sitting to one side of your legs and swinging your feet around to the front with bent knees to prepare for Rolling Like a Ball.

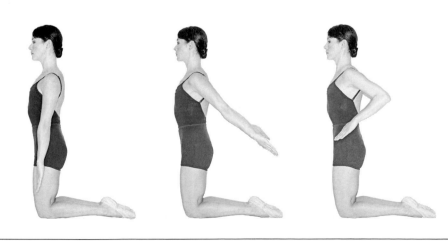

tones arms, legs, and buttocks,
opens chest and shoulders

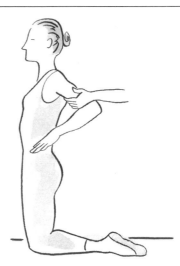

do

- Keep your legs *sewn together* tightly with your pelvis pressed forward to maintain a sturdy base from which your back can stretch.
- Use your breath to fuel your movements. Make sure you are creating imagined resistance.
- Keep elbows reaching for each other and arms squeezed tightly to your sides throughout.

don't

- Do not allow your shoulders to creep up around your ears.
- Do not allow your elbows to drop even 1 inch as you bend your arms.

modification: Perform the exercise standing in the Pilates stance with weight toward the balls of your feet. Glue your inner thighs together throughout.

progression: Perform the sequence in the Pilates stance, balancing on the balls of your feet. Heels and inner thighs are glued together throughout. You may lower your heels after each repetition.

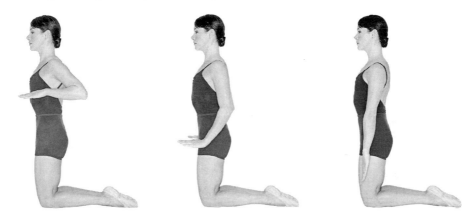

THE BREATHING

goal: To expand your lungs and increase your breathing capacity.

step by step

Transition from Crisscross by lying back and lowering your feet to the mat.

1. Lie on your back with your knees bent, hip-width apart, and feet flat on the mat; keep your heels almost directly under your knees. Stretch your arms straight up toward the ceiling, keeping your back flat and your shoulders pressing down into the mat.
2. Inhale as you simultaneously press your arms down and roll your hips up off the mat.
3. *Imagine a sling underneath your back and bottom hoisting you upward.*
4. Maintain your inhalation for a count of 5 as you press the backs of your arms into the mat and deepen the scoop in your powerhouse.
5. Press your pubic bone to the ceiling and your heels into the mat, *as if digging cleats into the ground.* This creates oppositional stretch for the fronts of your hips and thighs.
6. At the count of 5, begin slowly rolling down through your spine, reaching your arms forward and up until you have returned to your starting position.
7. Complete 3 to 5 repetitions. End by rolling up to a seated position. Straighten your legs out on the mat in front of you for the Spine Stretch with Arm Circles.

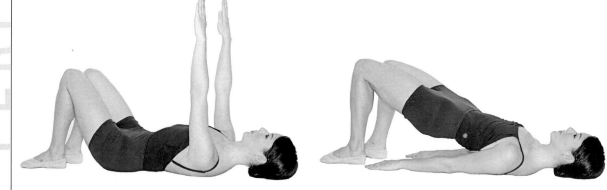

strengthens legs and buttocks,
stretches thighs, and flattens belly

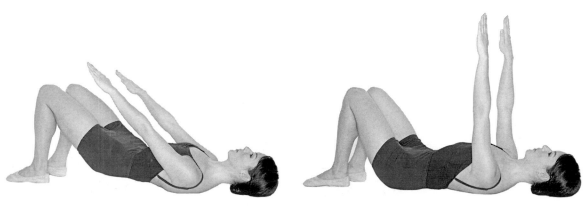

do

- Work to create imagined resistance as you press your arms through the air.
- Press the backs of your arms into the mat to help open your chest and shoulders.
- Engage the back of your neck, reaching the crown of your head away from your bottom as you roll down to create more length in your spine.

don't

- Do *not* allow your lower back to arch as you roll up. Press through your heels and curl up off the mat one vertebra at a time.
- Do not allow your knees to roll out or in. They must remain perfectly still throughout.

modification: Leave out the arm movements and simply roll your hips up off the mat, opening your chest and holding for as long as you can. Work up to 10 seconds.

progression: Increase the length of time that you can hold your inhalation.

SPINE STRETCH WITH ARM CIRCLES

goal: To increase the stretch of your spine and length of your waistline with each repetition.

step by step

1. Sit up tall with your legs extended on the mat and open to shoulder width.
2. Extend your arms straight out in front of you and flex your feet, *as if you were pressing your heels into the wall across the room.*
3. Inhaling, pull your navel deep into your spine as you sit taller, *as if the crown of your head were pressing up through the ceiling.*
4. Bring your chin to your chest and exhale as you begin to round down into a tight curl forward, *as if you were squeezing the last bits from a tube of toothpaste.*
5. When all the air has been squeezed from your lungs, begin a slow inhale as you reverse the motion of the exercise, rolling up, *as if constrained by a wall behind you.*
6. Exhale as you return to your tall seated position, with your arms extended in front of you.
7. Inhale and raise your arms up as high as possible without lifting up in your shoulders. Feel your waistline lift with the movement of your arms, *as if expanding in your center like a flexible pipe.*
8. Grow taller as you exhale, opening your arms (keep them in your periphery) and pressing them down to your sides with resistance, *as if swimming upward from the bottom of the ocean.*
9. Complete 3 to 5 repetitions. End by bringing your feet together and drawing them into your body. Take hold of the insides of your ankles in preparation for the Open Leg Rocker.

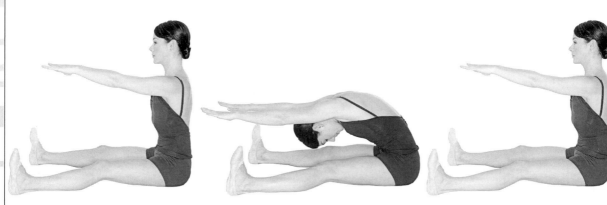

tones arms, legs, and bottom,
stretches hamstrings,
tightens waistline

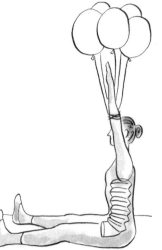

do

- Stretch the crown of your head up toward the ceiling and your shoulders down your back.
- *Imagine pressing your lower back and hips against a brick wall for stability.*
- Stay engaged through your legs and buttocks to increase the opposition to your spinal stretch.

don't

- Do not lean backward as you roll up. Keep your weight pitched slightly forward of center.
- Do not initiate the roll up with your head. Begin lifting from your powerhouse and let the head be the last piece to come up.
- Do not roll knees in as you stretch forward. Pull your toes back toward you as you go.

modification: "Soften" your knees to ease into the stretch forward.

progression: Add the arm movements from Rowing from Chest (p. 140).

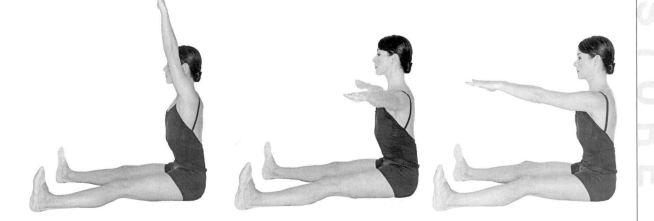

STOMACH MASSAGE III

goal: To stay lifted and light in your lower back throughout movements.

step by step

Transition from the Open Leg Rocker by bending your knees (keeping them open) and bringing your feet together, resting your toes lightly on the mat.

1. Sit balanced on your tailbone with your knees open just past your shoulders and bent into your chest, and with your toes resting lightly on the mat. Your arms are reaching up for the edge of the ceiling, but keep them inside your knees.
2. Inhale and lift out of your waist and the crown of your head, looking past your fingertips.
3. *Imagine you are balanced on a balance beam.*
4. Exhale as you simultaneously stretch your legs up and twist your upper body to follow one arm back. Keep your forward-reaching arm still as you "sweep" your opposite arm back, powering the twist from your center, *as if chopping a tree behind you.*
5. Inhale as you reverse the twist pulling your knees back into your chest and lightly touching the mat with your tippy-toes. Repeat on the other side. Complete 3 to 5 sets. End by rolling over onto your stomach to prepare for the Double Leg Kicks.

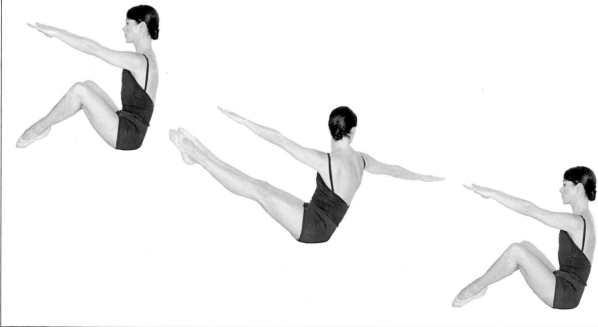

strengthens abs and legs,
stretches back muscles

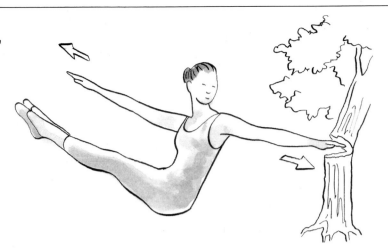

do

- Bring your chest up and forward to meet your legs as you draw your knees in.
- Keep your legs light by focusing on lifting with each twist.
- *Imagine balancing books on your head,* as you perform the sequence. *Keep pressing up on the books* to stay long in the neck.

don't

- Do not allow your knees to fall open. Maintain control with your inner thighs, *as if holding a ball between your knees.*
- Don't drop your feet as you bend your knees. Try to pull your knees back in toward your shoulders with control.

modification: Perform only the twisting portion of exercise. Keep your knees bent and feet flat on the floor or on tiptoe.

progression: Perform the entire exercise balancing on your tailbone. When your knees are bent, your toes remain lifted off the floor.

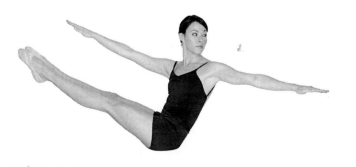

CHEST EXPANSION

goal: To increase your lung capacity and lengthen waistline.

step by step

Transition from the Low Back Stretch by rolling up to sit on your heels and then lifting your bottom up to a kneeling position.

1. Kneel on your mat with your legs hip-width apart, buttocks tight and arms reaching forward of your body.
2. Inhaling, pull your powerhouse in deeply and press both arms back with resistance, as far as you are able, lifting your chest in opposition to your elbows without allowing your ribs to stick out.
3. *Imagine you are the figurehead on the prow of a ship.*
4. Maintaining your inhalation turn your head to look right, then center, then left, and then center again before slowly exhaling and releasing the tension in your arms.
5. On the next repetition, begin the head turns by looking left first. Alternate with each repetition.
6. Complete 4 to 6 repetitions (or 2 to 3 sets, a set being one time looking right then left and one time looking left then right).

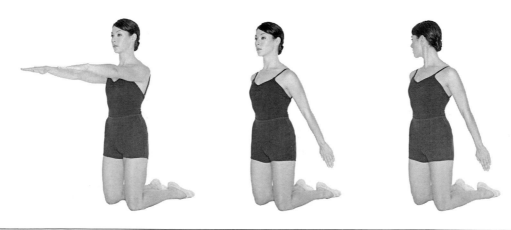

stretches neck, shoulders, and
chest, tones arms and buttocks

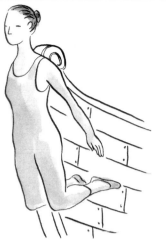

do

- Use control when turning your head from side to side to really accentuate the stretch of your neck muscles (*do not* push the stretch to the point of strain!).
- Engage your legs and buttocks throughout to create a sturdy base from which to move.

don't

- Do *not* allow your head to tip backward as you turn it side to side. Keep growing taller through the crown of your head and lengthening the back of your neck.
- Do not allow your back to arch as you press your arms back.

modification: Simply complete steps 1 to 3, leaving out the turning of the head. Concentrate instead on increasing the amount of time you are able to sustain your inhalation and expand your chest.

progression: Add a thigh stretch to the sequence by leaning your whole body backward in opposition to your arms as they reach forward. Do not put strain on your knees or break at your hips.

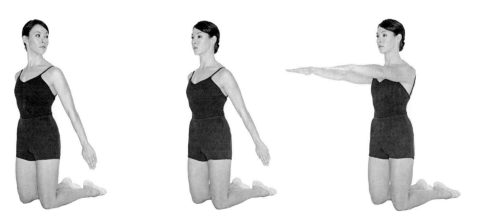

Finding Flexibility

Flexibility to some is an elusive concept and is likely the most neglected aspect of physical fitness. Flexibility decreases risk of injury, increases blood and nutrients to joints, decelerates joint degeneration, increases physical efficiency and performance, boosts neuromuscular coordination, and reduces muscle soreness. What's not to love? But most people believe that flexibility is either something you have or you don't. Not true. In fact the keys to finding flexibility are in the way you train your muscles to respond when called upon and how consistently you request them to work to their potential. The better practiced you are at a particular exercise, the greater chance you will have to obtain flexibility from performing it.

Finding Flexibility is a great way to help you increase both your mental and your physical range of motion. Your very commitment to achieving flexibility is a strong factor in achieving it. Proper breathing control is also key to a successful stretch. Proper breathing relaxes and warms by increasing blood flow and helps automatically remove lactic acid and other by-products of exercise. The most important thing to remember about achieving flexibility is that it requires strength to do so safely and efficiently, so no sloppy or haphazard movements allowed. Use *Your Ultimate Pilates Body Challenge* principles to achieve the best stretch you can get throughout your workout.

note: The Tantalizing Ten exercises are shown on the road map to indicate their placement within the new series. The instructions in the following pages pertain to the new Finding Flexibility exercises. I have slotted the new movements into the places I deem appropriate to keep the proper rhythm and flow of the matwork. In Pilates you are never in one position for too long and in keeping with that philosophy and its related cardio results, I have sewn each new exercise into the fabric of the Tantalizing Ten as seamlessly as possible. Instructions on each page will transition you from exercise to exercise. Remember to stay focused on your goal of increasing your flexibility without disregarding the strengthening aspects of each exercise. In order to find the balance in your body between flexibility and strength you must capitalize on the competence of your powerhouse.

road map

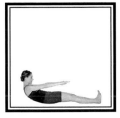

roll up
beginner

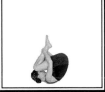

rolling like a ball
beginner

the tree
intermediate

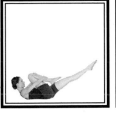

single leg stretch
beginner

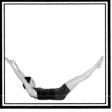

double leg stretch
intermediate

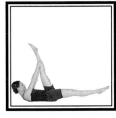

single straight leg
stretch
intermediate

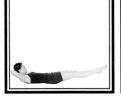

double straight leg
stretch
advanced

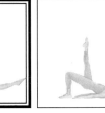

crisscross
advanced

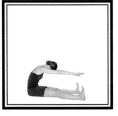

shoulder bridge
advanced

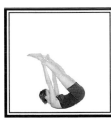

single straight leg stretch

spine stretch
forward
intermediate

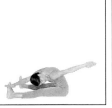

open leg rocker
intermediate

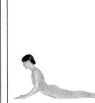

the saw
intermediate

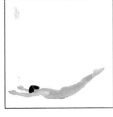

swan prep
intermediate

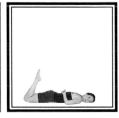

swan dive
advanced

double leg kick
advanced

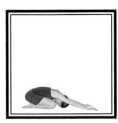

low back stretch

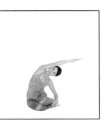

mermaid
intermediate

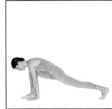

front split
intermediate

T H E   T R E E

goal: To lengthen your back and waist.

step by step

Transition from Rolling Like a Ball by releasing your ankles and grabbing the underside of one leg, stretching the other long on the mat in front of you.

1. Sit tall with one leg outstretched on the mat and the other leg bent into your chest; support your bent leg with layered hands. Hold the underside of your leg and not behind the knee.
2. Engage your powerhouse and lift your foot 1 inch off the floor.
3. Inhale as you straighten your leg to the ceiling, and exhale as you bend it again. Repeat this 3 times, growing taller with each movement.
4. On the last lift, leave your leg reaching for the ceiling and walk your hands to your ankle. Lift in your waist, *as if cinched in a corset,* and bring your chin to your chest, exhaling.
5. Using a deep scoop in your powerhouse to control the movement, slowly lean back until the back of your pelvis is touching the mat and your leg is straight to the ceiling.
6. *Imagine your leg is an oak tree.* Do not allow your supporting leg, *the root,* to lift up.
7. Using your hands to lightly support you, exhale as you walk them down your leg and press your spine down into the mat vertebra by vertebra. Maintain control from your powerhouse throughout.
8. Reverse the movement and walk yourself back up your leg, without allowing it to move. Lift up and forward into a tall seated position (as shown).
9. Repeat steps 4 to 6 three times. On the last repetition, stay tall, bend your knee, and switch legs. Finish by switching legs again, but this time slowly rolling your back down to the mat in preparation for the Single Leg Stretch.

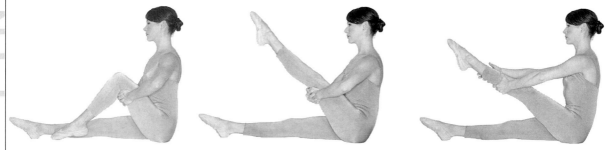

strengthens abs and lower back,
tones arms

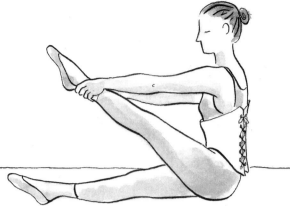

do

- Maintain wide, lifted elbows throughout to work the backs of your arms.
- If need be, sacrifice a bit of your straight leg by allowing it to "soften," but never sacrifice the lengthening of your back.

don't

- Do not lock your elbows or sink into your shoulders as you roll back.
- Do not drop your body weight down. Control the movement from your powerhouse.
- Do not grip with the front of your thigh. Try to maintain a slight turn out in the hip (as in the Pilates stance) to engage more of your buttocks muscles.

modifications: Perform steps 1 to 3 to help gain flexibility. As you feel more confident in your form, add on another step, one at a time. You may also keep a slight bend in your knees throughout the sequence.

progression: On your last repetition of step 7, lie down with your arms pressing into the mat by your sides. Do 3 leg circles in each direction, then climb back up the tree.

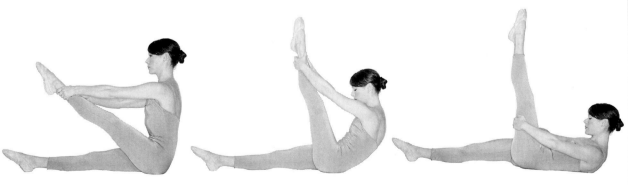

SHOULDER BRIDGE

goal: To stay absolutely still in your "standing" leg.

step by step

Transition from Crisscross by lying back onto the mat with your arms long by your sides and lowering your feet to the mat.

1. Lie on your back with your knees bent and feet planted firmly, with your heels almost directly beneath your knees. Knees and feet should be pressed together tightly.
2. Inhale, scooping your powerhouse and curling your tailbone up off the mat. Make sure you are engaging your buttocks by pushing through your feet.
3. Continue to inhale as you peel your spine up off the mat, vertebra by vertebra. Don't allow entire sections of your back to come up at once.
4. Exhale at the top and really sink your abdominal muscles deeper into your spine as you press your pubic bone to the ceiling.
5. *Imagine there is a hoist around your hips suspending you in mid-air.*
6. Stretch one leg out on line with your bent knee and reach for the opposite wall through your pointed foot.
7. Inhale and kick that leg to the ceiling without moving any other part of your body.
8. Now flex your foot and stretch, *as if you were trying to touch the ceiling.*
9. Lower your leg with resistance, *as if it were attached to a spring from the ceiling.*
10. When your heel nears the floor, point your foot and kick back up with precision and control.
11. Perform 3 to 5 kicks and then place your foot on the mat to switch legs. Complete 3 to 5 kicks with the other leg and then roll your spine down to the mat, vertebra by vertebra, stretching your arms even farther forward to help lengthen the movement.
12. Slide your feet farther away from your bottom and roll yourself up to sitting. Sit tall with your legs straight and open shoulder-width to prepare for the Spine Stretch Forward.

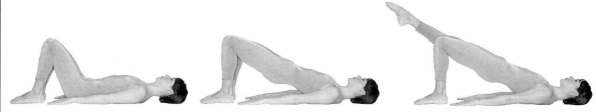

FINDING ADVANCED FLEXIBILITY

firms arms, legs, and buttocks

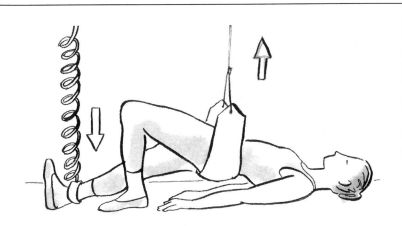

do

- Use your leg *like the lever of a car jack,* rising in your hips with each depression of the leg.
- Keep pressing the backs of your arms and shoulders deeply into the mat.
- Press through the entire sole of your foot to feel your bottom working.
- *Imagine the kicking leg begins under your rib cage and stretches through the front of your hip.*

don't

- Do not allow your bottom to drop even 1 inch as you perform the exercise.
- Do not allow supporting leg to roll in or out. Press through the foot to stabilize its position.
- Do not allow your tummy to stick up. You should be able to see your hips past your tummy.

modification: Practice rolling your pelvis up and down with your knees and feet squeezed together while still maintaining proper form and opening the fronts of your hips.

progression: After your last kick up, and while holding the lifted position, perform 3 bottom lifts trying to touch your pointed toe to the ceiling with each lift.

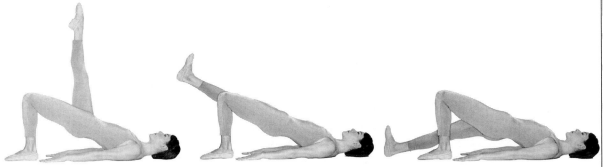

T H E   S A W

goal: To remain firmly anchored in your lower body, allowing your upper body to stretch freely.

step by step

Transition from the Open Leg Rocker by bending your knees and bringing your feet together on the mat. Release your ankles and straighten your legs out in front of you.

1. Sit up as tall as possible, with your open legs extended wider than hip-width apart and stretch your arms out to your sides, *as if you were reaching out to touch both sides of the room at once.* Keep your hands within your sight line. Flex your feet, pushing through your heels.
2. Inhale, drawing your powerhouse in and up your spine as you twist from the waist to your left. Stay evenly balanced, pressing the bones of your bottom down into the mat beneath you.
3. *Imagine you are buried in sand and are able to move only from just above your hips.*
4. Exhale as you round your head down to your left knee, reaching your right hand past your baby toe, *as if your hand were sawing off your baby toe.* Reach your other arm in opposition.
5. As you stretch down, deepen your exhalation by pulling your belly in opposition to your reaching hand, *as if being pulled back by a sling around your waist.*
6. When you have exhaled completely, inhale and begin drawing your body upward into the starting position, stretching the crown of your head up, *as if it could go through the ceiling above.*
7. Repeat the sequence to the right, exhaling deeply as you stretch your head to the right knee. *Imagine diving down into a pool as you round your head to your knee.*
8. Your opposite arm can remain lifted throughout the sequence to increase the oppositional pull.
9. Complete 4 sets. End by bringing your legs together and twisting your upper body to one side to place your palms on the mat. Roll onto your stomach with your hands under your shoulders to prepare for the Swan Prep.

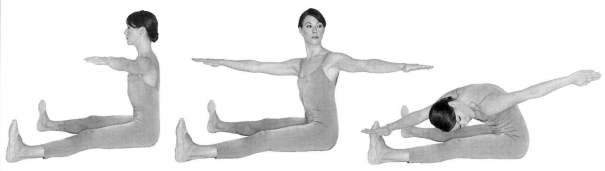

cleanses lungs, tones
arms, and tightens waistline

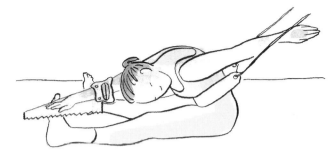

do

- Stabilize your hips to stretch by pulling your tummy up and away from your stretching arm.
- Remember to roll up to your starting position each time before twisting to the other side.
- Think of filling your lungs as you lift up and inhale, then *wring them out,* as you twist and exhale.
- Initiate rolling up from your powerhouse. Your head should be the last piece to come up.

don't

- Do not allow knees to roll in as you round. Make sure your big toes point toward the ceiling.
- Do not scrunch up in your neck as you round. Lengthen through the crown of the head.
- Do not twist from your shoulders and arms. Lengthen and twist from your waistline.

modification: Perform the exercise without raising your arms. Place your hands on either side of the leg you are rounding over and use your palms to support your upper body.

progression: Perform the exercise allowing your body to "bounce" with every sawing motion of your arm. Do *not* push yourself to the point of strain; these are *controlled* pulses to further stretch already warm muscles. Continue to pull your tummy in opposition to the stretching arm.

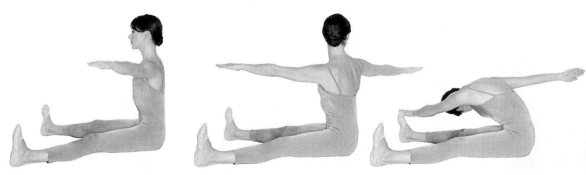

S W A N   P R E P

goal: To create stretch up the front of the body and warm back muscles.

step by step

1. Lie on your stomach with your palms pressing into the mat directly beneath your shoulders. Squeeze your legs together tightly. Actively press them—and your pubic bone—into the mat beneath you.

2. As you inhale, draw your navel up into your spine and begin straightening your arms. Lifting as high as you can without causing pain in your lower back. Keep your chest lifting and your neck long. *As if you were being lifted by marionette strings.*

3. Exhale and bend your arms, slowly lowering yourself back down to the mat while simultaneously stretching forward from your chest. Keep squeezing your buttocks and inner thighs together to support your lower back!

4. Do this stretch 2 to 3 times to warm up your back muscles then move on to Swan Dive if ready. Or lie flat with your arms bent behind back to prepare for the Double Leg Kick.

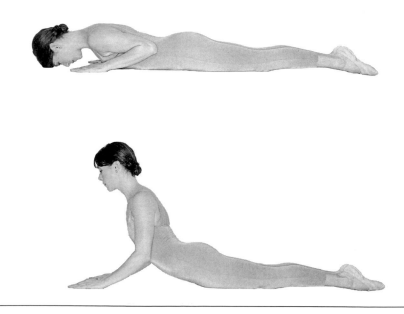

tones arms and firms buttocks

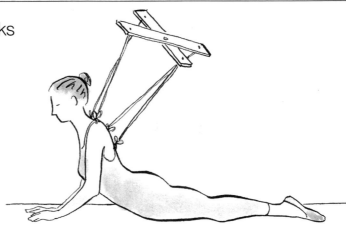

do

- Press through heels of hands to connect to side body.
- Pull powerhouse up to support spine.

don't

- Sink into low back.
- Do *not* drop your head back.

modification: From step 1 simply practice drawing navel up into spine and off mat. Repeat 5 times.

progression: On your last lift try rocking forward and lifting the legs behind you, then come back up by pressing into your palms. Try 2 to 3 rocking Swan Preps (see photo below).

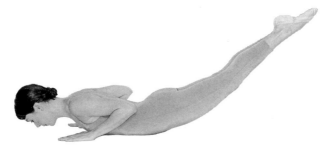

S W A N   D I V E

goal: To massage the front of your body without allowing your legs to come apart.

step by step

1. Perform the sequence for Swan Prep, and on the last stretch upward, with your chest lifted to the ceiling, release your hands and exhale, rocking forward onto your breast bone with your arms extended in front of you, palms up, and your straight legs lifted behind you.

2. *Imagine that you are diving forward to catch a beach ball.*

3. With the same momentum, inhale and rock back, lifting in your chest, and *imagine throwing the ball back over your head.* (Keep your arms and legs straight throughout the rocking motion.)

4. Keep rocking back and forth, inhaling on the back and exhaling on the forth.

5. *Imagine you are a giant ink blotter trying to absorb as much ink front to back as possible.*

6. Do a maximum of 6 repetitions, and then bring your palms back down to the mat and sit back onto your heels to release your lower back.

7. Hold this Low Back Stretch for one or two breaths, then stretch back out onto your stomach with your arms bent behind your back to prepare for Double Leg Kicks.

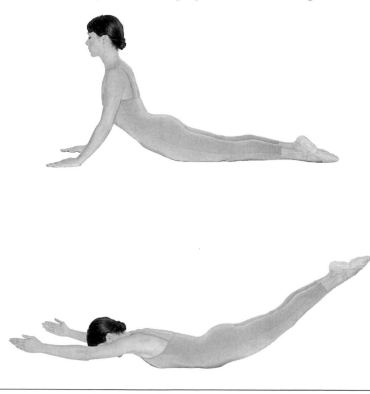

firms powerhouse,
stretches front and
back of body

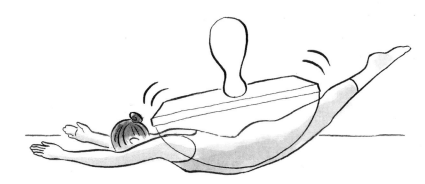

do

- Remember to engage the muscles of the powerhouse throughout to protect your lower back.
- Keep your heels *glued tightly together* for the entire sequence.
- Breathe dynamically during this exercise to create power for the movements.

don't

- If it hurts . . . STOP!
- Do *not* throw your head back and forth as you go. Lift from your chest and lengthen the back of your neck to secure the weight of your head.
- Do not lock your elbows or sink into your shoulders as you press up.

modification: Open your palms wider than shoulder-width apart. Also allow your legs to stretch long behind you, without squeezing them together but still actively pressing the tops of your feet and pubic bone into the mat beneath you.

progression: Reach back and take hold of ankles, rocking back and forth from powerhouse.

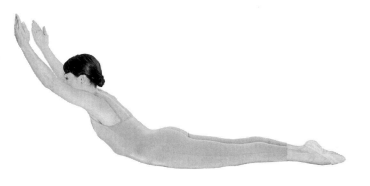

M E R M A I D

goal: To remain long and lifted on both sides of your waist.

step by step

Transition from the Low Back Stretch by rolling up to sit on your heels.

1. Sit on your right buttock with your legs bent to your left, knee over knee and foot over foot. Use your left hand to secure your ankles as close to your bottom as possible.
2. Inhale as you stretch your right arm up alongside your ear. Press shoulder down in opposition.
3. Exhale as you lean to your left, lengthening your right side. Wrap your arm over your head and try to touch your left ear. Keep your opposite elbow open and arm muscles engaged.
4. Inhale as you reach your hand toward the left wall. Lift your body back up to center.
5. Maintaining your inhalation, change arms by lowering your right arm straight down as you bring your left arm straight up and overhead. Place the palm of your right hand flat on the mat, as far as you can reach without collapsing and exhale all your air as you lean out over your right arm, allowing your arm to bend while still maintaining the lift in your waistline.
6. Use your powerhouse to avoid collapsing your right side, *as if stretching high over a cactus.*
7. Press your palm deeper into the mat, tighten your powerhouse muscles, and inhale to lift your body back up to center in one swift movement, switching arms and repeating steps 2 through 6.
8. Complete 3 to 5 repetitions on your right buttock and then switch sides. Finish by pushing up off your palm and lifting your body up to kneeling to prepare for the Front Split.

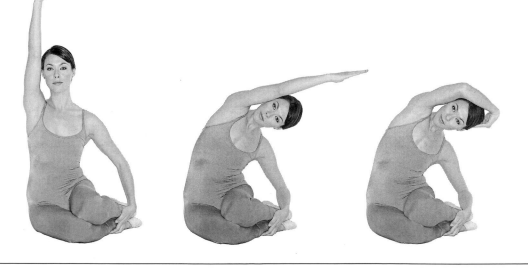

increases lung capacity,
tones arms and legs

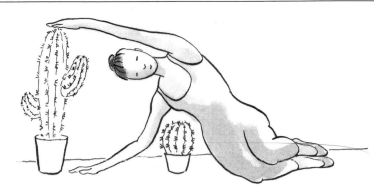

do

- Keep your supporting hand, the one on the mat, in *front* of your shoulder at all times. Do *not* lean to it if it is behind you, or you might damage your shoulder.
- Stay as long in your waist as possible to allow your arms to move freely.

don't

- Do not throw your arms. *Imagine they are moving like the pinions of a windmill.*

modification: Instead of knee over knee, allow your top leg to rest on the mat. Hold the knee or shin and perform steps 1 to 3 only.

progression: This is a *superadvanced* progression. Working with the utmost control, move your supporting hand farther away with each repetition (*always* keeping it in *front* of your shoulder line).

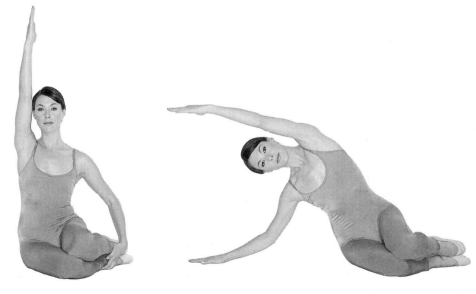

FRONT SPLIT

goal: To stay lifted in your powerhouse and light on your knees.

step by step

1. Kneel on your mat with your knees together and tummy tight. Open your arms if needed for balance. With one foot, take a giant step forward and lean your body forward placing your hands, or fingertips, down on the mat on either side of your foot. Make sure your front heel is directly beneath your knee. Your back leg should be stretched open past 90 degrees.

2. Curl your back toes under you and press the mat away with your palms to deepen your powerhouse connection.

3. Inhale and straighten your back knee up off the mat without moving forward or back in your body, *as if locking the hinge of a joint.* Make sure you are still lifted in your tummy and lengthening through the back of your neck. Stretch the crown of your head in opposition to your heel.

4. Lengthen more through the front of your hip by tightening your buttocks. Exhaling, release the stretch by returning your knee to the mat and uncurl your toes.

5. Without moving your hands, inhale as you straighten your front leg keeping your chest as close to the leg as possible without dropping your weight onto your thigh.

6. *Imagine being lifted in your center by hoist from the ceiling.* You may bow your head to your knee and relax your neck for a count of 3.

7. Exhale as you return to the forward starting position. Repeat steps 2 to 5 and then return to kneeling with knees together to switch legs.

8. Complete 2 sets on each side, alternating legs.

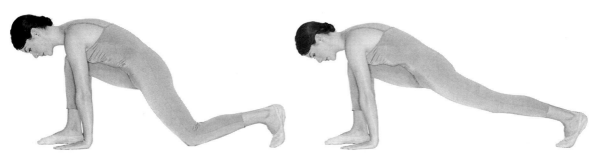

opens lower back, firms legs, improves balance

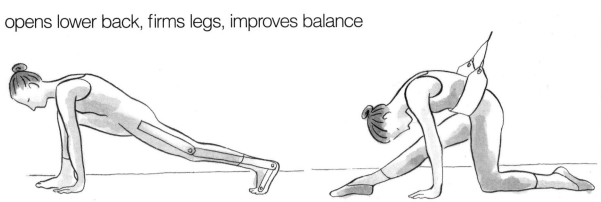

do

- Try to keep the sole of your front foot firmly pressing into the mat throughout the sequence.
- Keep "standing" weight into your front heel to engage your buttocks.
- Allow your straightened leg to be "weightless" by lifting in your powerhouse.

don't

- If this exercise hurts your knees . . . leave it out.
- Do not allow your head to hang down. Lengthen through the crown of your head.
- Do not grip or hyperextend your knees. Maintain length through your hips and thighs.

modification: Practice the stretch of step 1 only.

progression: From the position of step 1, lift your hands up off the mat and layer them behind the base of your head and lift your upper body to an upright position. Perform the rest of the steps in this position. (You will need to "bow" down to your knee when straightening your front leg.)

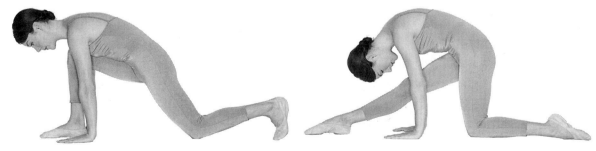

The Invisible Workout®

We all know the idea behind a microwave oven is heating from the inside out, even if we don't know the exact mechanics of how it works. Think of your powerhouse the same way. When we originate every action from our powerhouses and allow the energy to radiate out to our arms and legs, we work stronger, safer, and more efficiently.

Using the Pilates principles already identified, we'll now look at four "core" motions or actions integral to our everyday life: standing, sitting, carrying, and lifting. You may think you know how to stand and how to sit . . . possibly even correctly. The difference is that as you begin to perform these seemingly mundane motions consciously, with correct alignment, you get an all-day lengthening and strengthening workout.

We'll start by looking at the dos and don'ts of these four actions. Then I will show you how to integrate this knowledge into invisible daily exercises during the hours we are all most active. While there are no set numbers of reps or sets, be mindful to work your body evenly and consciously enough to feel the work. The movements are subtle, but effective, and will serve to raise your body's awareness. Eventually, connecting to your body in this way will be second nature, so that as you stand in line, you can firm your bottom, or as you sit at your desk you can target your obliques. Your boss will think you're deep in thought—and you are! It's just that you are thinking about your powerhouse.

Before we begin, however, it's a good idea to reiterate some of the non-negotiable principles discussed earlier. Remember that there are some form elements that, whatever you are doing, must be in play for you to be working safely, strongly, and efficiently. Following are the four non-negotiables to keep in mind as you move through your Invisible Workout®.

the non-negotiables

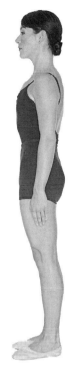

Your powerhouse is always engaged: "In and Up." Beginning without this step is like starting to drive without pressing down on the gas pedal. You might be able to roll along for a while, but it will only be downhill.

Your chest is always lifted. Not only is this better for your spine, it's better for your cardiovascular and circulatory systems, too. If you are hunching, you aren't breathing at capacity. Open up your chest and create the square footage of a mansion to house your lungs.

Your spine is a straight line, down through your crown. Rounding the back, hunching the shoulders, all of these things exert an enormous amount of pressure on your vertebrae. Keeping your spine in a straight line is like taking the kink out of your garden hose. It keeps the energy moving freely through your entire body.

Your weight is distributed evenly. Shifting your weight, whether it's into one leg, or into the back of your sofa or car seat, will always affect the natural curvature and abilities of your spine. Remaining mindful of your evenly rooted stance, whether you are sitting at your computer or rummaging through boxes in the basement, will ensure your body is working safely and at its maximum potential in everything you do.

Note: As we created the artwork for this section—and it was the first time my secret shape-up tips were let out of my head into the world at large—I realized some of the things I do to stay fit while standing on a city curb waiting for a walk sign may be a bit awkward for the self-conscious reader. The way I look at it is this: I'd rather look a bit foolish for a few minutes in front of people I'll never see again to look fabulous in front of people I really care to impress. You're not hurting anyone, you're helping yourself and—who knows?—you may just inspire someone else. After all, a few pliés on a street corner have got to be better than a doughnut on the hips any day, right?

S T A N D I N G

Most of us spend our time in line shifting miserably from foot to foot. And if we work long hours on our feet, we long for nothing more than to come home and put them in a warm bath before we have someone else massage them. How can we ameliorate the discomforts that plague us? Properly engaging our powerhouses will take the strain from our lower backs, arches, and knees, while giving us perfect poise and posture.

As you stand in line . . .

do

- Keep lifting through the arches of your feet so that all your weight isn't sinking toward the floor.
- Keep your shoulders rolling down and back, away from your ears, and your chest lifting up.

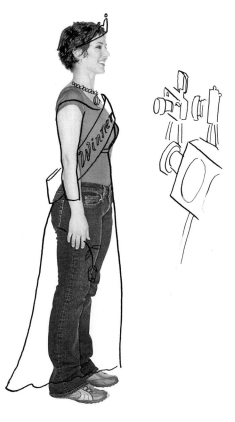

imagine: You are poised on the red carpet, in front of hundreds of photographers.

- Don't lock your knees. Allow a slight bend in your knees to help you to remember to engage your buttocks.
- Don't keep your weight on one leg only. Stay balanced by anchoring both feet firmly to the floor.

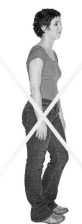

challenge

Standing-in-Line Swan Lake. As you stand in any interminable line—say, at the post office or the grocery store take the opportunity to work your powerhouse, buttocks, and legs with mini-arabesques. Standing with hips and feet facing forward, draw your powerhouse in and up and then lift your leg gently up and back, without moving your torso forward or tightening the muscles of your lower back. Repeat on both sides till you get to the front of the line.

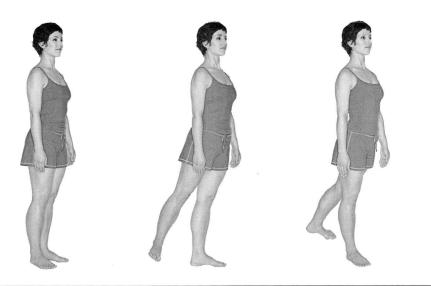

STANDING

As you stand at the photocopy machine . . .

do

- Lengthen your waist until it feels like it is higher than the copier.
- Pull up through your inner thighs and tighten your buttocks.

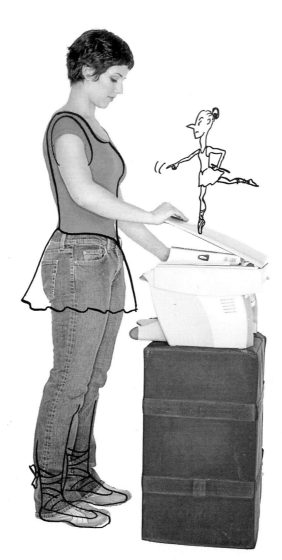

imagine: You are preparing to have your posture judged by the grande dame of the studio.

- Do not lean, thinking of this as wasted time. You're on an exercise break!
- Don't let the weight of your head pull you forward over the machine. Stay lifted and long in your neck.

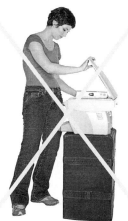

challenge

The 2 × 4 for 9 to 5. As you stand at the elevator or photocopier, you can tighten and tone your legs, buttocks, and abs. Standing in Pilates stance, draw your powerhouse in and up and rise gently up to the balls of your feet. Lower as in a plié to a count of 4. Keep your tailbone firmly tucked throughout. Lower your heels to the floor and stand up, drawing together your inner thighs. Reverse the movements.

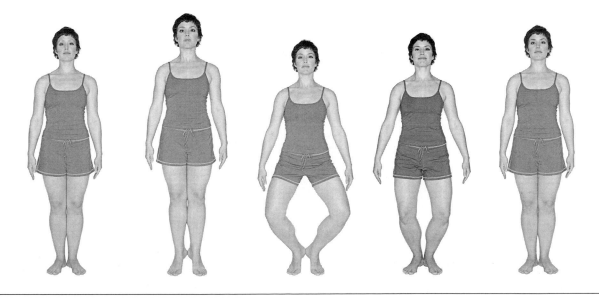

As you stand on the bus or subway . . .

- Keep your knees soft to absorb the rattles and rolls of the bus's movement.
- Keep your tailbone lengthening away from the crown of your head, and your waist cinched, while breathing freely and fully.

STANDING

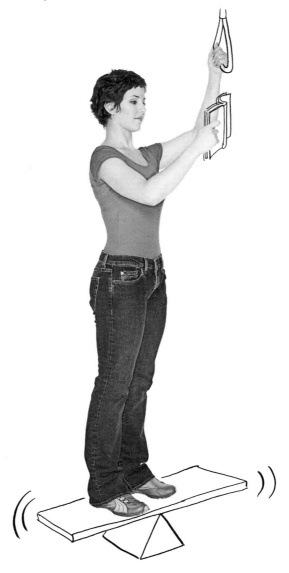

imagine: You are standing on a seesaw or surfboard, trying to find the balancing point.

- Don't hang off the straps or lean into the poles. Keep lifted and supported through the strength of your powerhouse. Use straps solely for balance.
- Don't hang your head down to read standing up. Hold the item you are reading at eye level to keep your neck long and supported.

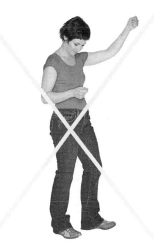

challenge

The Commuter Re-Creator. As you hold the strap on the bus or subway do some pliés to re-create a shapelier silhouette. Taking a Pilates stance, draw your powerhouse in and up, and then gently bend the knees without bringing your heels off the floor. Keep your tailbone lengthened and the crown of your head lifting. Go low. Go slow. Then stand, bringing inner thighs together.

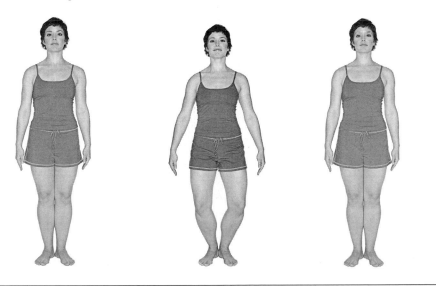

S I T T I N G

Neck strain, back pain . . . sitting without an engaged powerhouse can lead to a laundry list of nagging ailments. We need to know what it means to lift from our powerhouse and create internal columns of muscle to support us. Once we familiarize ourselves with, and master, this proper form then we can engage our surrounding muscles without risk of injury and increase our core strength with every move we make.

As you sit in commuter traffic . . .

do

- Raise your car's seat back to a 90-degree angle to ensure your straight spine.
- Use your grip on the wheel to help lift your upper back out of your waist, instead of lifting your shoulders up around your ears.

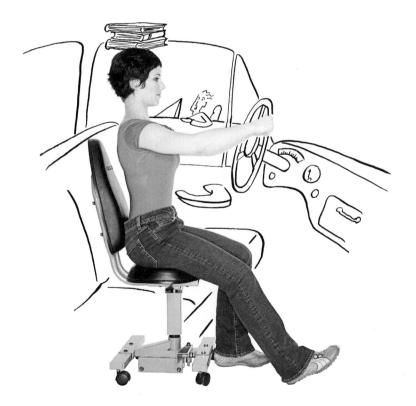

imagine: You are in a posture class at charm school with books balanced on your head.

- Do not sink into your lower back.
- Don't let your legs roll inward or drop out to the side. Keep your knees hip-width apart.

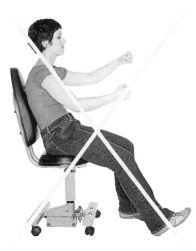

challenge

The Red Light Re-Shaper. As you sit at yet another red light, pull your powerhouse in and up, engage all the muscles of your buttocks, and then push down gently on the steering wheel, *as if you were going to lift yourself off your seat.* Hold for a count of 5 and then release. Repeat until the light changes.

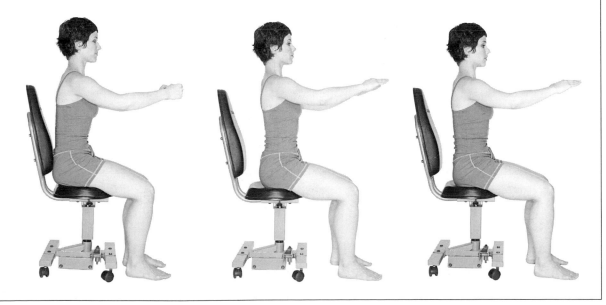

As you sit at your computer desk . . .

do

- Keep your chest lifting and pitch forward slightly from your hip bones. You should be able to feel your sitz bones on the seat. (Your "sitz" bones are the bones on the bottom of your bottom.)
- Keep your feet firmly planted at a right angle, to absorb some of your body's weight.

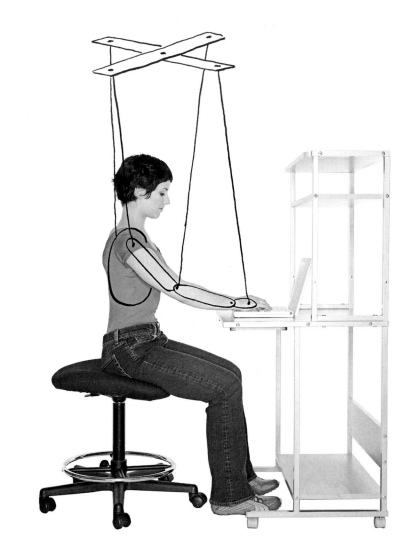

imagine: You are a dangling marionette with strings that suspend you from the ceiling.

- Don't sit in one position for more than 20 minutes. Get up, stretch, and shake out your limbs.
- Don't let your bottom curl underneath you. Keep lifted in your lower back by placing a hard cushion behind you—or get a chair with no back at all!

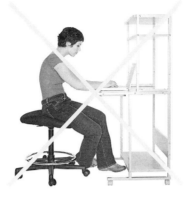

challenge

The Air Chair. Place your hands, palms down, against the arms of your chair, then press down hard enough to lift your buttocks off the seat of the chair 1 to 2 inches and hold yourself in mid-air for a count of 3. Make sure you are not sinking into your shoulders, your tummy is pulled in, and your knees are squeezing tightly together. (If your chair has no arms, place your hands on either side of the seat and press with the heels of your hands until you have raised yourself into the air.) Now try picking up your feet off the floor. Take care not to slip on arms of chair.

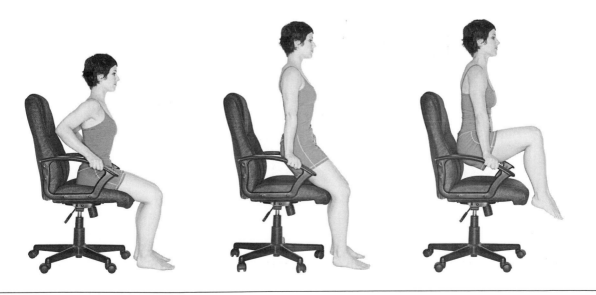

As you watch TV . . .

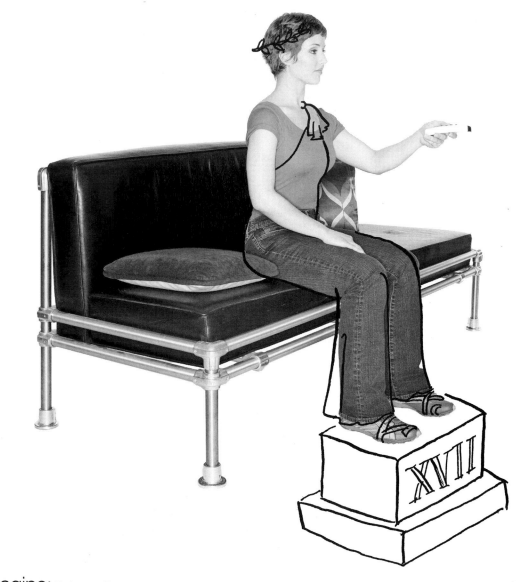

do

- Use the time productively for stretches on the floor or over a physio ball or hard pillow. Try to stretch your back in the opposite direction of your seated posture.
- Get up and move around during commercials or sit on the edge of your seat with perfect posture.

imagine: Being a Greek sculpture. Maintain the form in which you wish to be memorialized.

- Don't become so engrossed in your program that you lose your body awareness.
- Don't slump down in your chair or sofa with your tailbone curled under you. Better to lie flat on the floor than to sit with an incorrectly rounded spine.

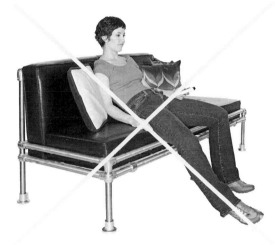

challenge

Must-Knee TV. As you sit at the front of your sofa or chair, press the heels of your hands down on the front edge of the sofa to help you lift in your waistline. Alternate lifting your knees as high as you can without losing your form, and hold them up as long as you can. Try to extend your leg then bend it in again. Remember this is a powerhouse exercise, so stay lifted and don't round that back! Higher ratings for a double-leg lift.

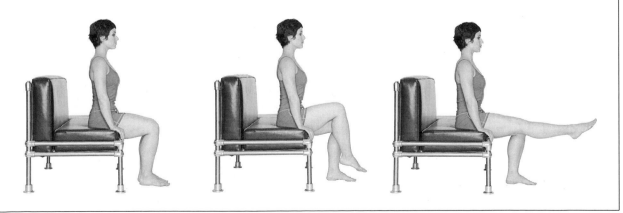

C A R R Y I N G

We've all experienced the aching back that can come from lugging bags of groceries, suitcases, or our little ones from place to place. Here I'll show how too many of us sabotage our bodies and what we can do to ensure a future of swinging our children—and grandchildren—with abandon and filling our grocery carts without worrying about carrying everything into the house.

While carrying your bag to work . . .

do

- Balance the weight of the bag by shifting upper-body weight to equal it on the opposite side.
- Stay lifted in your waistline to help take some of the weight off your shoulder and elbow joints.

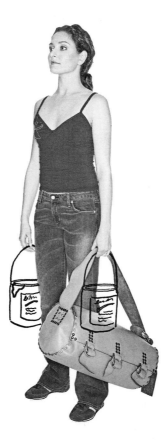

imagine: Carrying buckets of paint, keeping them evenly balanced so you don't spill a drop.

- Don't put your free hand in your pocket because it makes it all the more difficult to create the opposing weight with your opposite arm.
- Don't slouch; the added weight of the bag is hard enough on your muscles.

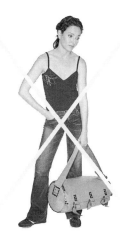

challenge

Biceps-Bag Curls. A new take on a classic curl. Make sure never to allow the arm to extend fully, so that you keep the muscle long and engaged, and avoid locking the elbow joint. Use long slow movements to get the most resistance from this exercise. Depending on the bag handle, these can be performed single- or double-armed.

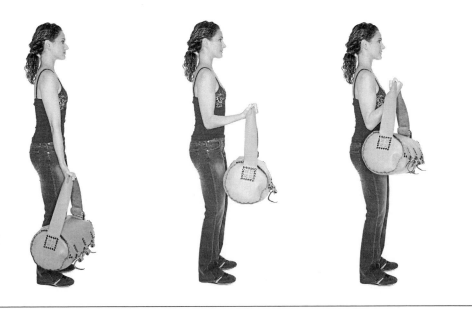

As you carry your shoulder bag around town . . .

do

- Try to balance your shoulders out by pressing the nonengaged shoulder down and back.
- Stay lifted in your waistline to allow the shoulders to relax and even out.

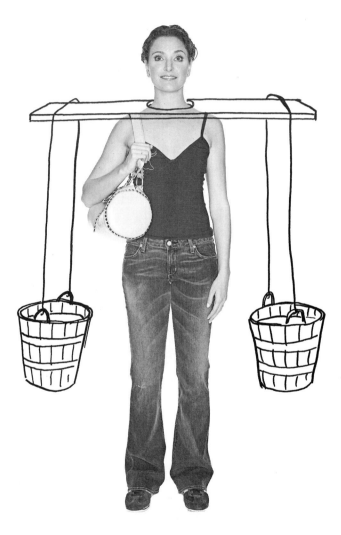

imagine: A yoke across your shoulders, keeping them pressed down and evenly balanced, allowing the muscles that run along the side of the neck to the shoulder to stretch.

- Don't allow your body to lean away from the bag in an attempt to compensate for the bag's weight.
- Don't always carry your bag over the same shoulder; be sure to switch sides frequently.

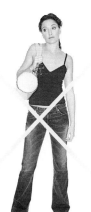

challenge

Shoulder-Bag Shoulder Circles. While circling one shoulder, keep the other shoulder blade pulling back and down. Be sure to fuel this motion from your shoulder blades and emphasize the downward motion of the circle. Don't hunch your shoulders up around your ears.

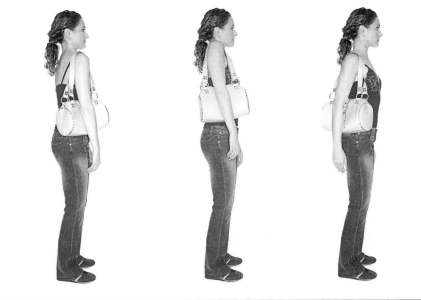

CARRYING

As you carry your kids . . .

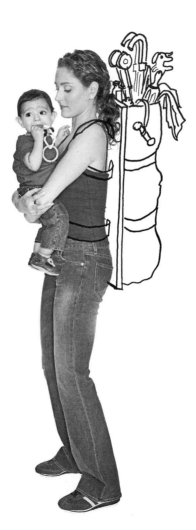

do

- Switch sides often to avoid overdeveloping and shortening the muscles of one side only.
- Try to keep the child slightly toward the front of your body when carried on your hip to allow the shoulder girdle to remain straight (so your spine is not constantly twisted toward the baby).

CARRYING

imagine: Having your back pressed against a rucksack and keep the back of your hips and shoulders pressed evenly to it.

- Don't lock your knees when standing still with the baby on your hip to avoid putting too much pressure on the hip and knee joints.
- Don't use only one arm to support the child, try to engage both sides of the body and stay square and lifted at the same time.
- Don't let your shoulders roll forward. Keep pulling your shoulder blades down and together.

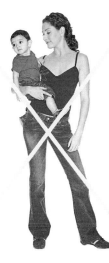

challenge

The Toddler Twist. Standing with your feet wider than shoulder-width apart and your knees bent in a semi-squat, hold your darling to the front of your body. Twist side to side, staying lifted in your waist to work your oblique muscles. Make sure to keep your knees soft and anchor your feet to the floor. Do not allow your knees to move as you twist.

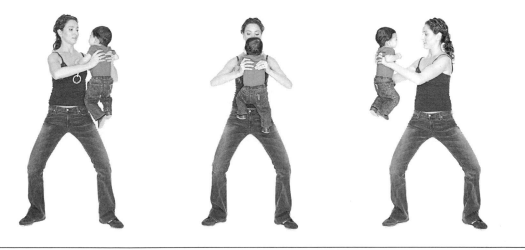

CARRYING

L I F T I N G

Boxes, furniture, children . . . By this time, most of us have a sense of what not to do when lifting a heavy object. We know that lifting must originate from a properly engaged powerhouse or begin with bent knees to ensure the safety of our backs, knees, and shoulders. Here I'll show you how to make the most of these common movements—so they're not only safe but also effective.

As you lift your kids up to the jungle gym . . .

do

- Squat to your child's height before you begin the lift.
- Shift the balance of your weight to your heels and initiate the movement by pushing the ground away.

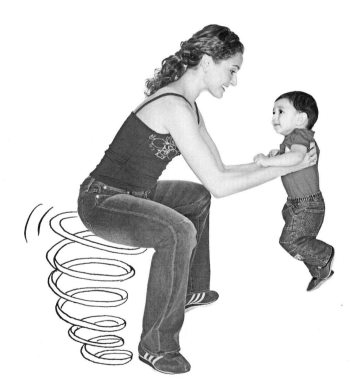

imagine: You are sitting onto a heavily coiled spring as you squat to pick up your child. Use the energy of the spring to lightly bounce back up to standing.

- Don't scoop your child up with one arm.
- Don't pick your toddler up while twisted or with the majority of your weight in one leg. Make sure that you are facing your child and use slow, controlled movements.

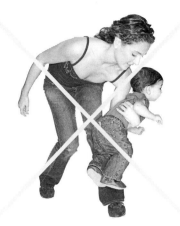

challenge

The Stooping-to-Conquer Squat. Say, for example, when you got home you put your groceries on the floor, rather than on a counter before unpacking them. How can you make the putting-away process a workout? Squats, of course! Keeping your body in one line, bend your knees to squat down to pick up one or two items. Make sure your powerhouse is engaged and your weight is firmly in your heels. Then, on an exhalation, push the ground away as you lift up, engaging the muscles of your legs as well as your bottom.

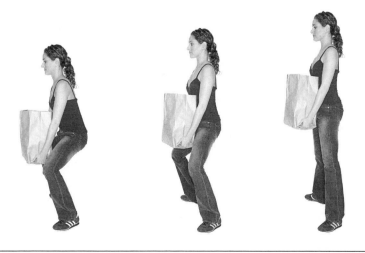

LIFTING

191

As you hoist that box up onto the shelf . . .

do

- Originate the motion from your center—keep pulling your powerhouse in and away from the box.
- Take the majority of the box's weight in the heels of your hands to engage the muscles of your trunk, and not your arms and back.

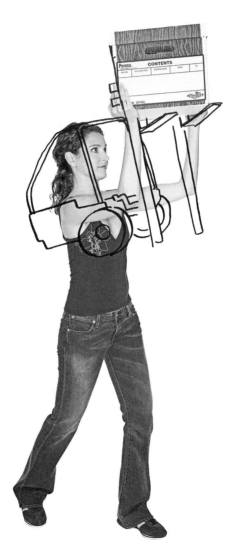

imagine: You are a forklift, slowly and deliberately raising the load to its destination.

- Don't hold your breath! Use your breath to reinforce correct movement; inhale as you pick the box up and exhale as you lift it overhead.
- Don't try to get the box overhead using momentum. Keep your movements steady and controlled.

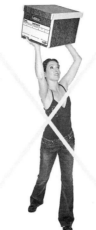

challenge

The Overhead Olympics. Before you lift that (manageably weighted) box over your head to place it on a shelf, bend your knees to give your bottom, abs, and legs a workout. Then with control, stretch (your torso first and arms last—work the larger muscle groups first!) upward to place the box on its shelf. Bonus points will be given if you can rise up on your toes at the end of the motion. Then, slowly lower your heels down.

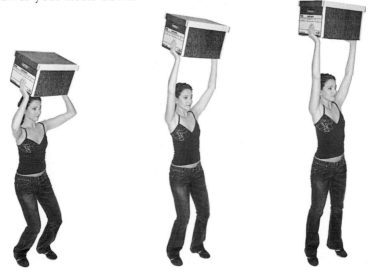

LIFTING

As you lift furniture or luggage (one-handed lifting) . . .

- Balance your weight to accommodate the weight of the lifted object.
- Bend at your knees, not your waist, to release your lower back.

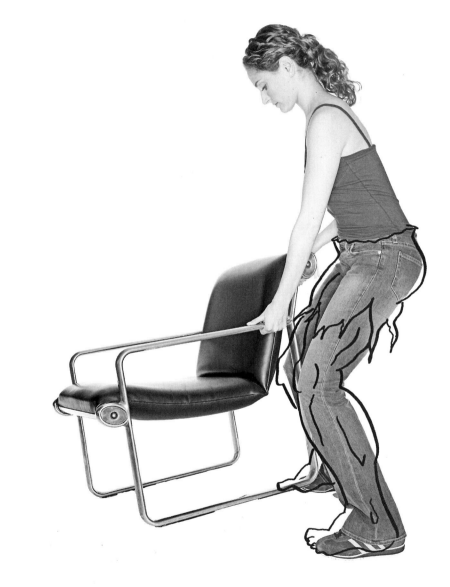

LIFTING

imagine: You've engaged your leg muscles so powerfully that they are ripping through your pants.

- Do not lock your knees to support the weight of the lifted object. Use your legs and bottom to support the weight of the lift.
- Don't allow your shoulders to roll forward, or you will be lifting from your upper back and not using the strength of your powerhouse.

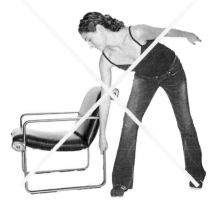

challenge

The Triceps Triage. As you are moving through your day, take the opportunity to make your furniture your gym with triceps dips. Standing with your back to a sofa or sturdy chair, place your hands on its arm with your fingers pointing toward you. Move your body away to a 60-degree angle. Gently bend your elbows, so you are doing a reverse push-up. Keep your body in one line so that your abs and legs keep working too.

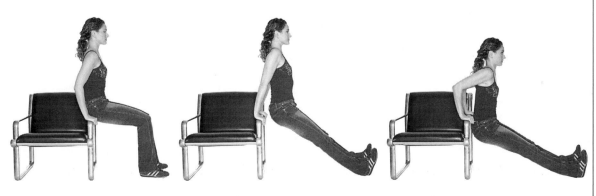

chore challenges

Learn to make the world your gym! How about stretching your Achilles tendons by using the edge of the curb as you wait for the light to change? Or try performing the Roll Up as you get out of bed in the morning. Find specific ways you can use the world around you to lengthen, strengthen, and tone your Pilates body. Here are some examples to get you started.

Look Forward to Housework

Pilates principles while mopping? Why not? Standing in one spot with your feet parallel, turn your body to the side and stretch the oblique muscles as you push out, then strengthen them as you lift yourself back to an upright position. How far can you stretch without moving your feet, resting your weight on the mop handle, or putting pressure on your knees? Once you've mopped the maximum circumference you can reach, move to a new spot and repeat. Remember to switch sides often so you don't overdevelop one side.

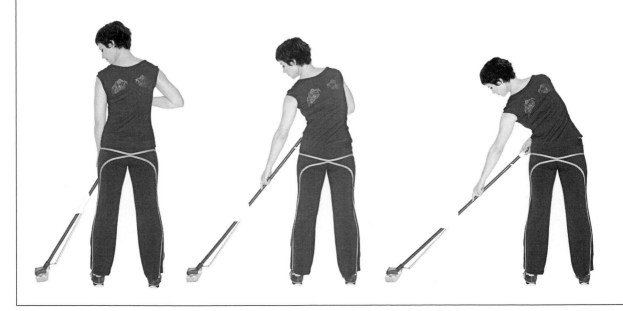

The Couch-Potato Workout

Sit on the front edge of your couch or chair with your legs at 90-degree angles and hip-width apart. Place a tea towel or dish rag flat on the floor in front of your toes. Without allowing your heels to lift off the floor begin by stretching your toes out over the towel and then curling your toes to gather the towel up. When you've gathered up the entire towel perform the exercise in the reverse until the towel is flat in front of you again. This stretches and strengthens all the muscles of your feet and is especially great for arthritis sufferers.

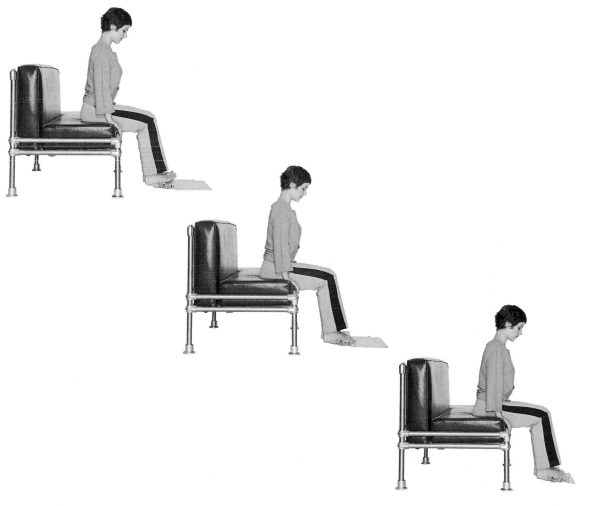

Your New Baby and You

Let's face it, as much as you'd like to, you can't spend all day sitting on the sofa admiring your baby. Sometimes you need to get out and about, so put him or her in your stroller and hit the road! As a new mom, I am now acutely aware of the terrible posture I see in today's stroller pushers. As you walk or run with your stroller, think about your Pilates principles and how you put them into effect on the treadmill. Don't lean into or over the stroller handles. Use the resistance of the stroller to help you lift your chest. Lengthen your waist and push the ground away from you to engage your powerhouse muscles. Gripping the handles too tightly forces too much energy into your arms and shoulders, so try a light grip or even an open-handed push when in a safe, nontrafficked area.

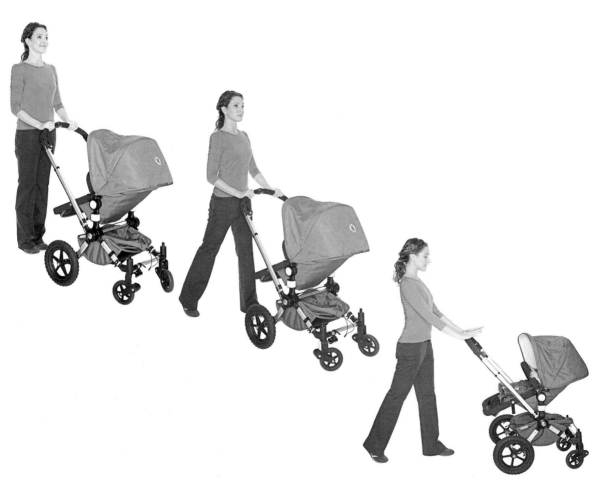

Pilates in the Snow

When shoveling, make sure that your front foot faces the direction of whatever you are going to be working on shoveling. Really bend your front knee to "get under" what you are lifting and don't allow your back foot to lift from the ground. Make sure not to stand so far from what you're shoveling that you need to lean out or stretch to reach it, as this forces the weight into your arms and shoulders and away from your powerhouse.

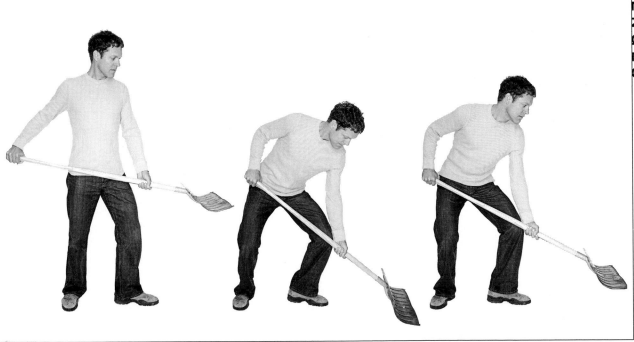

Pilates for the
Sports-Minded:
Super-Sizing Your Internal Super-Athlete

What turns an athlete into a super-athlete? Of course, there are hundreds of different factors, but the two constants I've observed are (1) super-athletes have an incredibly strong grasp of the essentials—they have a solid foundation on which to build, and (2) they never stop learning, never stop believing there is still room for improvement.

Tiger Woods is an excellent example of this kind of dedication and curiosity. Approximately two years into his professional career, he left his game to go back to basics. During that time, he completely revamped his approach to his swing. What was one of the things he chose to incorporate into his new education program? Pilates.

How can Pilates lower your par, power-up your serve, or take seconds off your slalom? The same way you've seen it maximize your gym routine and make housework or photocopying . . . well, if not a joy, at least an opportunity for awareness. Engaging your powerhouse throughout every motion will unleash energy and strength you never knew you possessed. The concentration and focus you've been fine-tuning during these last few chapters will allow you to follow through with maximum control and precision.

As you'll see, the exercises in this section have been specifically designed both to incorporate Pilates principles and to lengthen and strengthen those areas of the body commonly foreshortened or ignored while participating in various sports.

An example of the kind of foreshortening I'm talking about can most easily be seen in the sports that emphasize the use of the upper body—primarily because of various racquets and clubs—such as tennis and golf. Because players of these sports so often keep the majority of their focus on the side of their body that holds their club or racquet, their bodies tend to have foreshortened muscles on that side. These exercises will lengthen and strengthen these areas, enhancing much-needed stability and range of motion.

With skiing and snowboarding we'll also look at common problems and provide exercises to strengthen and lengthen the muscles that must work to give these athletes the global conditioning necessary for peak performance.

Before I begin, however, I think it's worth speaking again about those elements of Pilates form that remain non-negotiable.

the non-negotiables

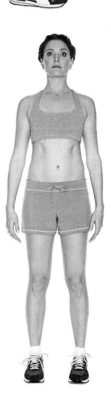

Your powerhouse is always engaged: "In and Up." "In and up" was the way Joseph Pilates described the main action of engaging the powerhouse. By pulling your abdominal muscles in and up, you are reminding yourself to lift your waistline, creating more room for circulation and a more secure stabilizing structure for your lower back.

Your chest is always lifted. Oxygen is the true unsung hero of any sport. Efficient breathing enhances all your movements, adding power and endurance to your craft. Joseph Pilates asked that full inhalations and exhalations be performed without fail. Given that, it is essential to keep your chest lifted to allow for the maximum lung expansion possible.

Your spine is a straight line. This is so, even with the understanding that as you hit an overhead smash or sink a long-distance hole-in-one there will be moments of curving, twisting, and bending. My point here is more that your head should always be working in tandem with your spine—not in opposition to it. Its weight should not be pulling you out of alignment or off balance.

Your weight is distributed evenly. There will obviously be numerous moments when weight shifts will be critical to ace your serve or traverse those moguls. For example, you might need to shift your weight into one foot to complete a serve or a swing or a hairpin turn, but as you take your Pilates body out into the world, you will learn to work with resistance and opposition so the rest of your body can compensate.

G O L F

do

- *Think of your club as an extension of your arms,* not something you grip. This will allow you to use the muscles of your torso more efficiently than just using your wrists and shoulders.
- Use the ground as a launchingpad, from which you can draw energy for your swing.
- Use your gaze as an extension of your twist.

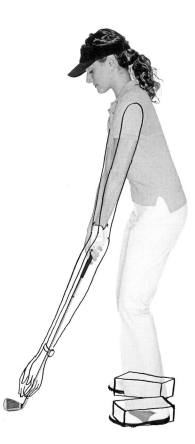

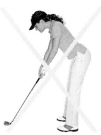

don't

- Don't round over your club from your shoulders. Lengthen from your waist.
- Don't follow your downswing down. Create opposition by lifting your body up as your club comes down; remember leverage.
- Don't tip your body forward. Keep your weight evenly distributed through the balls and heels of your feet.

Wrist Strengthener: Sandbag Lift

Whenever you introduce a piece of handheld equipment, one of the first things you're told is not to "break at the wrist." Easier said than done—and many of us haven't spent a lot of time working on our wrist strength, which is needed to avoid the break in that line. Here's an easy exercise I have my golf and tennis aficionados do to strengthen and tone the muscles of their wrists.

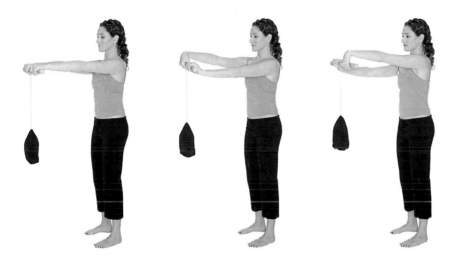

1. Tie a length of rope (floor to shoulder height) around the middle of a wooden dowel.
2. At the end of the rope, tie a sock or piece of cloth partially filled with sand or pennies.
3. Standing with your arms extended, straight in front of you at shoulder height, begin to turn the dowel, raising the sandbag. Make sure you are using only your hands and wrists to perform this movement; don't allow the elbows or shoulders to help the action.
4. *Imagine raising a sack of priceless diamonds from the bottom of the ocean.* Use control so that you don't lose them forever.
5. When the sandbag reaches the dowel, reverse the action. Make sure your shoulders stay down, and your powerhouse is engaged.

Other Great Wrist-Strengthening Exercises

Swan Prep (p. 162)
Mermaid (p. 166)

Kneeling Side Circles (p. 132)
Long Stretch (p. 120)

Lower Back Strengthener: Pilates Swimming

Bending over your tee incorrectly can be murder on your lower back—even when your form is correct. To strengthen these all-important muscles, I recommend this exercise.

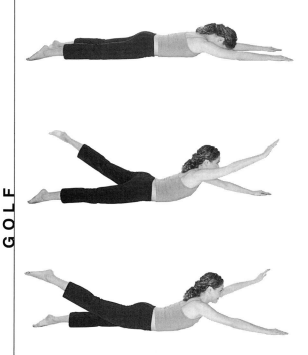

1. Lie on your stomach, completely outstretched on the mat. Reach your fingertips for the wall in front of you, and your toes for the wall behind.
2. Inhale and pull your navel up into your spine as you bring your right arm and your left leg up into the air simultaneously. Hold them there as you lift your head and chest off the mat as well. Remember to keep your powerhouse engaged to protect your lower back.
3. Holding your head and chest steady, switch your arms and legs.
4. *Imagine you are balancing on a tightrope* as you continue switching your arms and legs.
5. Keep your line of vision above the surface of the "water," without dropping your head back. Keep your arms and legs as straight as possible throughout the exercise, without allowing them to touch down to the mat.
6. Complete 2 to 3 sets (inhaling for 5 counts and exhaling for 5 counts equals 1 set) and then sit back on your heels to release your lower back.

Other Great Lower-Back-Strengthening Exercises

Spine Stretch Forward (p. 102)
Grasshopper (p. 130)

The Tree (p. 156)
Reformer Teaser (p. 122)

Side Lengthener: Standing Side Bends

As I mentioned earlier, many times athletes who use handheld equipment have unknowingly foreshortened the muscles on one side of their body—the side that manages their racquet or club is quite strong, pulling the muscles of their other side out of alignment. This simple side stretch will bring balance and flexibility to your body and your game.

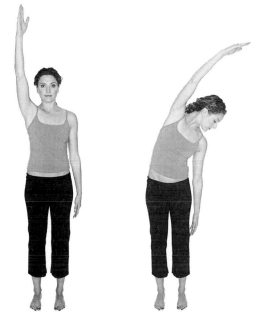

1. Stand with your feet parallel and raise your right arm toward the ceiling. Don't let your shoulder scrunch up near your ear.
2. Slowly lift and lengthen your torso as you bend to your left. Turn your head to look at the floor, increasing the stretch in your neck. Try to keep length in your left waist.
3. *Imagine you have a raw egg between your hips and rib cage and you don't want to crack it.*
4. Inhale to bend; exhale as you slowly straighten back up to center.
5. Repeat on the other side.
6. Complete 5 sets.

Other Great Side-Lengthening Exercises

Mopping (p. 196)
Crisscross (p. 100)

The Saw (p. 160)
Stomach Massage III (p. 150)

T E N N I S

- Keep your shoulders down to engage your middle back, adding power to your swing.
- *Think of your spine and legs as being spring loaded,* to avoid excessive pressure on your joints.
- Remember to keep your weight even, especially when you're reaching for a shot. Cultivate a sense of how your whole body is moving across the space.

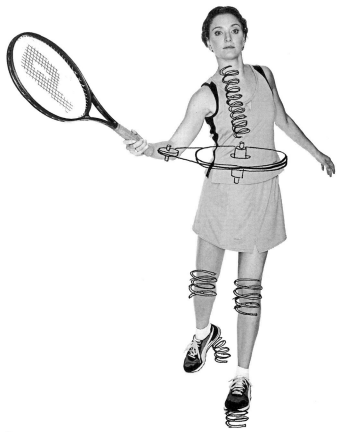

don't

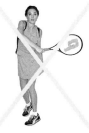

- Don't shorten the space between your ribs and hips when twisting. Stay long in your waist to access your powerhouse.
- Don't work only on the balls of your feet. Shifting your weight to your heels for a shot allows you to access the muscle power of your back body.
- Don't allow the momentum to be generated from your shoulder. Fuel your swing from your powerhouse.

Neck Strengthener

Most of us don't spend a lot of time thinking about toning our neck muscles, and yet almost all of us notice times of neck tightness, pain, and fatigue. This simple exercise will strengthen your neck so that it works to support you, whether you are lunging to return that seemingly impossible forehand volley or looking up to get the angle for a perfect overhead smash.

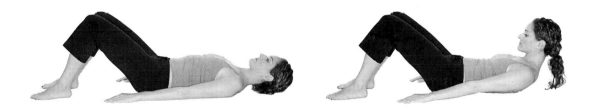

1. Lie flat on your back with the soles of your feet flat on the mat, about a beach ball's distance from your bottom.
2. Begin reaching your arms forward to pull your shoulders away from your ears. Then slowly lift your head, making sure to leave space between your chin and your neck.
3. *Imagine you are rounding your chin over a tennis ball.*
4. Hold your head up for a count of 3 breaths. Make sure your powerhouse is engaged and your back is flat.
5. Slowly lower your head.
6. Repeat 5 to 8 times.

Other Great Neck-Strengthening Exercises

Long Strap Circles (p. 126)   Chest Expansion (p. 152)
Double Leg Stretch (p. 94)   Pull Straps II (p. 142)

Hamstring Strengthener

Unevenly developed hamstrings can do a lot to pull the body out of alignment, throwing off your shots. Here's an exercise to strengthen and tone your hamstrings evenly, giving you the power to get to the ball in seconds and providing a strong foundation to support your stroke.

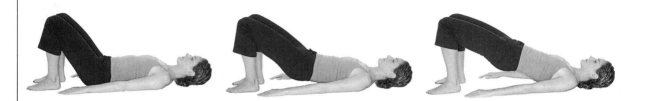

1. Lie on your back with your feet hip-width apart and your heels directly under your knees.
2. Engage your powerhouse and keep your neck long as you slowly lift your hips toward the ceiling and press the backs of your arms deeper into the mat.
3. Hold for a count of 5, keeping your hamstrings and buttocks engaged and your powerhouse pulled in and up.
4. *Imagine there is a red-hot branding iron underneath your bottom.*
5. Articulate your spine as you roll your back down toward the floor.
6. Complete 5 to 8 repetitions.

Other Great Hamstring-Strengthening Exercises

The Breathing (p. 146)   Long Back Stretch (p. 144)
Shoulder Bridge (p. 158)   Double Leg Kicks (p. 106)

TENNIS

Quadricep Lengthener/Single Leg Kicks

As always, everything works in unison. So, as we strengthen the hamstrings, it's important to lengthen our quadriceps, balancing the power of our legs. This stretch will allow your quads to release and lengthen, facilitating the strengthening and toning of your hamstrings.

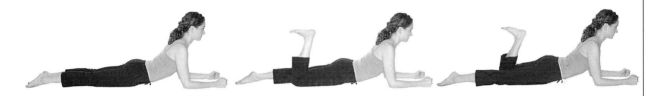

1. Lie on your stomach with the back of your legs squeezing together behind you; prop yourself up onto your elbows with your navel pressing up into your spine and your pelvic bone pressing firmly down into the mat.
2. Squeeze your buttocks and backs of your inner thighs together to support your lower back. Make sure that your chest is lifted so that you do not sink into your shoulders and back of your neck.
3. Your hands can be made into fists and positioned directly in front of your elbows. (If fists are uncomfortable place your palms face down on the mat.) Think of lifting your upper body away from the mat by pressing away from the elbows.
4. Lengthen your spine and begin by kicking the right heel into the right buttock with a double beat.
6. Switch and kick the left heel to the left buttock with a double beat. Straighten the opposite leg when it is not kicking. Do not let it touch back down to the mat in between kicks.
7. Remember to stay lifted in the abdominals by pressing away from the elbows.
8. *Imagine you are trying to tap yourself on the back with your foot.*
9. Complete 5 sets and end by sitting back on your heels to release your lower back.

Other Great Quadricep-Lengthening Exercises

Single Straight Leg Stretch (p. 96) Front Split (p. 168)
Grasshopper (p. 130) Balance/Control (p. 128)

TENNIS

DOWNHILL SKIING
do

- Access the twisting power of your powerhouse. Be fluid and dynamic. Keep your upper body (and belly button) square to the hill.
- Keep your upper body quiet. The counterrotation of your hips initiates your turn. *Imagine you are unscrewing your lower body out of your waist.*
- Keep your stance square—hips, knees, and feet in alignment. Knees should not roll in or out.

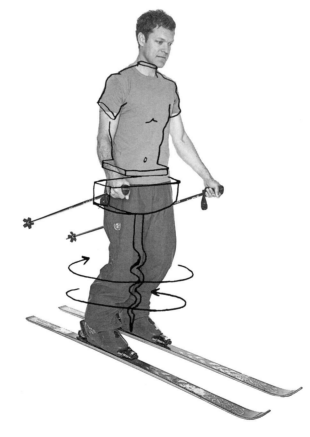

don't

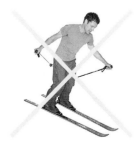

- Don't tighten muscles of your feet. Relax to facilitate weight shifting.
- Don't shift all the weight to your toes. Work through the entire foot to access muscles of both your front and back body simultaneously.
- Don't allow your gaze to drop. Your gaze should be about three turns ahead. It governs the direction of your body.

Oblique Strengthener: The Crisscross

As discussed, you're going to need the muscles of your side body to be both strong and flexible in order to give you the strength and range of motion you'll need to do some serious twisting. Here is an oblique muscle strengthener to help you maximize the power of your side body.

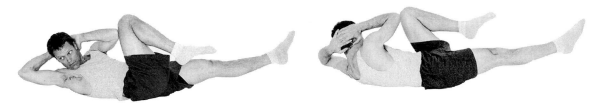

1. Lie on your back with your hands behind your lifted head and shoulders, and your knees bent into your chest.
2. Extend your left leg out long—about 6 inches off the mat—while twisting your upper body until your left elbow touches your right knee. Inhale as you lift. Make sure you are lifting from below your shoulder to reach your knee and not simply twisting from the shoulder socket.
3. Look back to your right elbow to increase the stretch and hold the position as you exhale. Make sure your upper back and shoulders do not touch the mat as you twist and hold the stretch.
4. Switch the position by inhaling and bringing your right elbow to your left knee while extending the opposite leg out in front of you. Hold the stretch as you exhale completely.
5. *Imagine twisting your body like a marshmallow being pulled into taffy.*
6. Complete 5 to 10 sets and then pull your knees tightly into your chest.

Other Great Oblique-Strengthening Exercises

Mopping (p. 196)
Mermaid (p. 166)

The Saw (p. 160)
Stomach Massage III (p. 150)

Oblique Stretch: The Chair Twist

As always, stretching is as important as strengthening. This stretch for the oblique muscles can be done anywhere you have a swivel chair and a little bit of time and energy to spare.

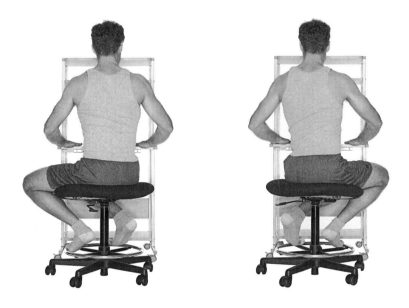

1. Sitting on the front edge of a swivel chair, place your hands, palms down, on your desk.
2. Ideally, your knees should squeeze together tightly and your feet should be lifted 1 inch off the floor. If this is not possible, modify by leaving the balls of your feet on the floor or footrest of the chair.
3. Without moving your chest from its lifted and straight forward position, begin twisting the chair from side to side, simultaneously stretching and toning the oblique muscles.
4. *Imagine you are wearing a heavy armor suit and helmet and are unable to move your upper extremities even 1 inch as you perform the twist from your lower body.*
5. Perform 10 to 20 rotations.

Other Great Oblique-Stretching Exercises

The Toddler Twist (p. 189)   Swan Prep (p. 162)
Mermaid (p. 166)   Stomach Massage III (p. 150)

Buttocks and Leg Strengthener: Leg Pull Down

In addition to your fully engaged powerhouse, strong, toned legs are a must for balance and support. This exercise works these all-important areas.

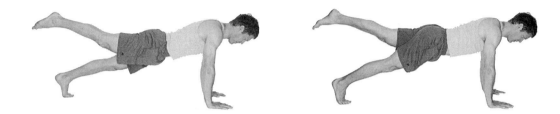

1. Place your hands, palms down, onto the mat underneath your shoulders and pull your navel up into your spine as you press yourself up into a push-up position.
2. Squeeze up the back of your legs and make sure your body is held in a straight line.
3. *Imagine you are a rod of steel from your head to your heel.*
4. Inhale as you kick one leg straight up off the mat behind you and pulse it twice in the air.
5. Exhale as you bring it down to the mat and switch legs.
6. Switch legs with each breath. Complete 3 sets.

Other Great Buttocks- and Leg-Strengthening Exercises
Shoulder Bridge (p. 158)   Gondola (p. 134)
Long Stretch (p. 120)   Standing Leg Press (to the back) (p. 136)

SNOWBOARDING

do

- Keep your center of gravity low—in your powerhouse—while remaining fluid in your legs.
- Angle forward from your knees and drive through each turn with your powerhouse as your engine.
- Remain quiet and open in your upper body *like the yoke of the Liberty Bell.*
- When you find you need to "monkey-hop" uphill for a few yards, let your powerhouse provide the momentum for the turns. Don't default to your hip flexors or quads.

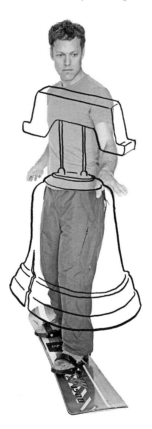

don't

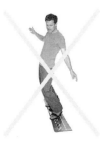

- Don't lock the joints of your leg to make the turns. Using your powerhouse takes more strength, but will keep you fluid.
- Don't default to your quads when you are working the toe edge of your board. Use your powerhouse to keep your weight centered.
- Don't default to your buttocks muscles to access the heel edge of your board. Keep weight in your heels, but use your powerhouse to center yourself.

Foot-Muscle Lengthener

No one wants a twisted ankle or foot cramp to derail their fun. This exercise is great for strengthening ankles while stretching the muscles and tendons of the feet.

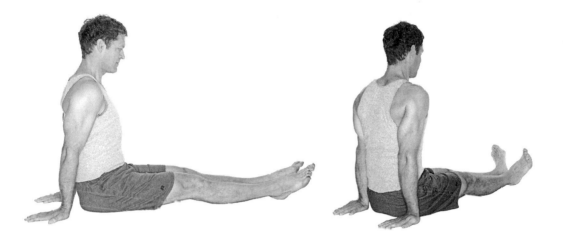

1. Sit on the floor with your spine lifted and your shoulders rolling down and back.
2. Lift up out of your lower back, as you engage your powerhouse.
3. Inhale as you point both of your feet as strongly as possible, then flex them as you exhale all of the air out of your lungs.
4. *Imagine you are trying to press an elevator button that is just out of reach—first with your toes, then with your heels.*
5. Complete 5 sets.

Other Great Foot-Muscle-Lengthening Exercises

Single Straight Leg Stretch (p. 96)   Shoulder Bridge (p. 158)
Standing Leg Press (to the front) (p. 136)   Front Split (p. 168)

Calf Strengthener

Strong calf muscles are a must for navigating snowy slopes. This exercise is great for strengthening these all-important muscles.

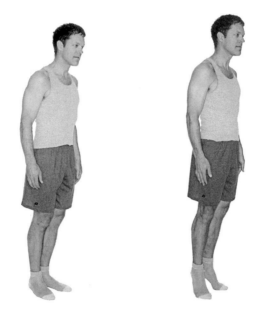

1. Stand in the Pilates stance; heels together, toes apart.
2. Engage your powerhouse as you inhale and slowly rise up onto your toes. Make sure your heels stay glued together.
3. Press your inner thighs together to engage your buttocks and hamstrings even more.
4. *Imagine you are gripping the winning lottery ticket between your heels and someone is trying to snatch it.*
5. Hold for a count of 3.
6. Exhale as you slowly lower yourself back down to the floor.
7. Complete 5 sets.

Other Great Calf-Strengthening Exercises:

Shoulder Bridge (p. 158)

Long Stretch (p. 120)

The 2 × 4 for 9 to 5 (p. 175)

Standing Leg Press (to the back) (p. 136)

Transverse Muscle Strengthener

Strong transverse muscles are essential for twisting, turning, and maybe even somersaulting on the slopes. This exercise will give you the confidence you need to perform with ease.

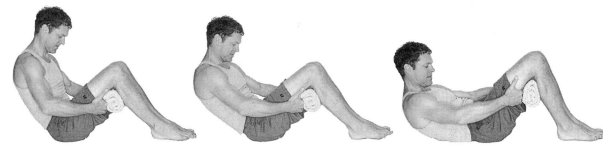

1. Sit with your knees bent and feet squeezing together, a beach ball's width from your bottom.
2. Place a thickly rolled towel behind your bent knees and squeeze to engage your hamstrings.
3. Using your hands on the underside of your thighs, inhale and begin rolling down toward the mat, placing each vertebrae down carefully as you go.
4. Stop when the bottom of your shoulder blades reaches the mat. Exhale completely as you deepen the scoop in your powerhouse.
5. *Imagine your stomach is a large bowl waiting to be filled with your favorite food.*
6. Inhale as you squeeze the towel tighter and begin rolling back up to a seated position.
7. Complete 5 to 8 repetitions.

Other Great Transverse-Muscle-Strengthening Exercises

Rolling Like a Ball (p. 90)   The Breathing (p. 146)
Single Leg Stretch (p. 92)   Stomach Massage III (modification) (p. 150)

challenge

Take your newfound awareness into a sports or outdoor activity that hasn't been discussed: riding, skateboarding, boxing, soccer, martial arts, rollerblading, cross-country skiing, windsurfing, surfing, and see what you discover. When you work with your Pilates principles, how does the sport change for you?

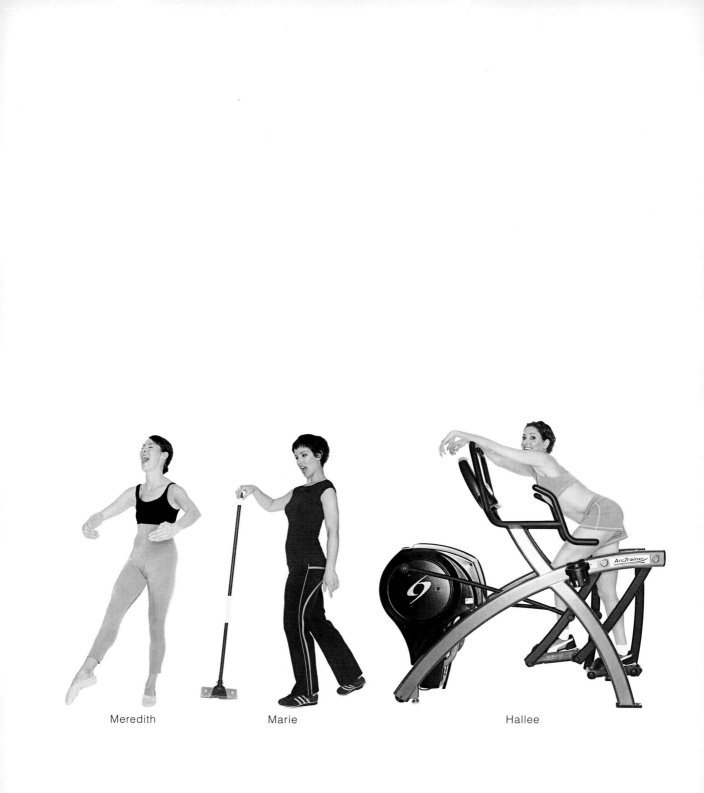

Meredith   Marie   Hallee

Thanks for your patience, prowess, and loads of laughs.

acknowledgments

Thanks to my Wonder Woman of an agent, Debra Goldstein; Frances "the Shark" Jones for her sublime writing flair while under the influence of caffeine; the supreme PR talents of Sarah Hall Productions, with personal thanks to the queen bee Sarah herself; to Marc Royce, whose artistry rivals the masters and humbles the saints.

Thank you to the superb stylings of Katy Robins; beauty aficionado Claudia Pedala; rock-steady illustrator Meredith Hamilton; my editor, Trish Medved, and the entire team at Broadway Books.

Particular thanks to Top Pilates Models: Hallee Altman, Meredith Sheppard, Marie Gruss-Sherr, and Chris Cady.

To Beth Boyd, Tedd Drattell, and the re:AB® crew for keeping the studio on its toes in my absence. It's a joy to work with you, and without you all this book would not have been possible. Thank you!

I would like to thank the following companies for the generous use of their superb clothing and accessories: Capezio, Danskin, Fit Couture, Marika, PANYC, Kara Janx @ 30 Van Dam, and Shiva Shakti.

Last but not least . . . to the Katzes, Schlachters, and Silers for always making their hearts my home and grounding me. I love you all.

To my second family, the Liebers, for their endless love, support, and generosity.

To Delia, for her patience, faith, and extraordinary care.

And to my mother for her courage, style, spirit, and kind, kind heart . . . I love, admire, and treasure you.

fitness resources

This is a resource list of talented professionals, outside the realm of Pilates, with whom I have collaborated and whom I would like to thank for their continuous support and great work. They have been instrumental in my physical well-being over the years. In the year following my pregnancy, they helped me to rediscover, reeducate, and re-create my former physical self. I recommend them highly.

- Gideon Orbach DC
  GideonOrbachdc@yahoo.com
  www.gochiropractic.com
- Shawna Cordell Fitness
  255 Center Street
  New York, NY 10013-3214
  (212) 925-7177
  www.shawnacordellfitness.com
- Stephen F. Oswald DC
  80 Fifth Avenue
  New York, NY 10011-8002
  (212) 924-2121
  www.drstephenoswald.com

- Shannon O'Kelly DC
  73 Spring Street # 207
  New York, NY 10012-5801
  (212) 334-3395
  www.networkwellnesscare.com
- Joel Kaye, MA
  physical health education
  (917) 400-4021
  JoelKaye15@yahoo.com

For more information on Brooke Siler and re:AB® Authentic Pilates, or to find an authentic instructor in your area, or to book a re:AB Pilates session, please visit our Web site at www.reABnyc.com.

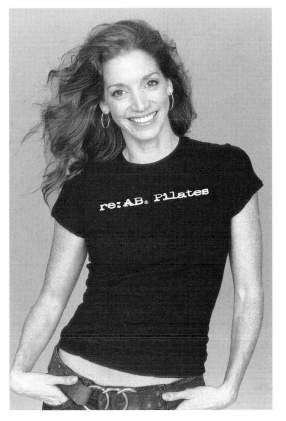

about the author

Brooke began her Pilates career in 1994 under the tutelage of Joseph Pilates's protégée Romana Kryzanowska. In 1997 she coordinated the creation and development of re:AB®, New York City's award-winning studio for Pilates. Committed to the idea that exercise is more than just physical exertion, Brooke has successfully brought her dedicated clients to new levels of fitness and personal satisfaction. Siler's unique methods of visual imaging and unswerving dedication to clients have earned her a position as one of the most sought-after personal trainers in the country, as cited by *Vogue* magazine. She is reshaping the landscape of the fitness world with a decidedly fresh and holistic approach to working out. Brooke is the master sculptor behind some of the most lithe and sleek physiques in Hollywood and on the runways.

In January 2000, Brooke's first book, *The Pilates Body* (Broadway Books), was published. Later that same year it made the *New York Times* bestseller list. *The Pilates Body* has been translated into seven languages and continues to break all sales records of titles in its field. Brooke's most recent publication, *The Pilates Body Kit,* is an audio CD series helping to bring Pilates into the homes of those unable to access an authentic studio in their area. September 2005 will mark the beginning of Brooke's long-awaited re:AB Authentic Pilates Teacher Certification program in which she will work to create top Pilates professionals who will carry the Pilates method forward to subsequent generations.

Brooke has been seen in dozens of national and international publications from *Vogue* and *Glamour* to *New York* and *People*. She has been featured on programs such as the *Today* show, *Entertainment Tonight,* Discovery Channel's *Home Matters, Ainsley Harriott, Fine Living,* and *The Main Floor,* as well as on NBC, ABC, CBS, NY1, VH-1, E!TV, and Fox News channels.

Based in her hometown of Manhattan with her husband and son, Brooke teaches workshops and lectures internationally.

For more info on Brooke please contact Sarah Hall Productions 212-529-1598 or the re:AB Pilates Studio at 212-420-9111 (www.reABnyc.com)

Brooke Siler

Invites you to visit

re:AB® pilates

authenticity. passion. purpose.

est. 1997

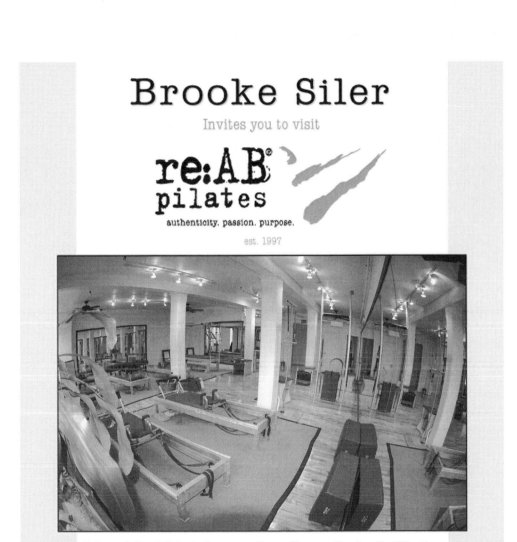

Private & Semi-Private Lessons · Group Classes · Teacher Certification

33 Bleecker Street, NY. NY. 10012
212.420.9111
www.reABnyc.com

Visit our Website to see Special Promotions for Readers of
YOUR ULTIMATE PILATES BODY CHALLENGE